PRIVATE PRACTICE IN NURSING

Development and Management

Charles J. Koltz, Jr., R.N., M.P.S.
Community Mental Health Nurse
Central Islip Psychiatric Center
Central Islip, New York

Aspen Systems Corporation
Germantown, Maryland
London, England
1979

Library of Congress Cataloging in Publication Data

Koltz, Charles J.
Private practice in nursing.

Bibliography: p. 237.
Includes index.

257 p.
ill. b. n.

1. Nursing—Practice. 2. Nursing—Practice—
United States. I. Title.
RT86.7.K64   338.4'7'61073   79-9311
ISBN 0-89443-158-7

Library of Congress Catalog Card Number: 79-9311
ISBN: 0-89443-158-7

Printed in the United States of America

1 2 3 4 5

For
My mother Eleanor
and
my father Charles
whose contributions were unselfishly given.
Without their support my nursing practice would not be.

Table of Contents

Chapter 4 — Assessment — The Basis for Determining
                 Community Needs..........................   51

    Community Assessment   51
    Community Needs   55
    Summary.....................................   57

Chapter 5 — Services Provided and Specialization   59

    Determining What Services To Provide...........   59
    Case Presentations.............................   72
    Summary.....................................   78

Chapter 6 — Professional Relations..........................   81

    About Public Relations........................   81
    Professional Relationships — New Roles   84
    Summary.....................................   97

Chapter 7 — The Professional Corporation....................   99

    Preparing for a Professional Corporation   99
    Summary.....................................   105

Chapter 8 — Promoting the Practice   107

    Publicity.....................................   107
    Summary.....................................   113

Chapter 9 — Model of a Private Practice.....................   117

    Impressions..................................   117
    Summary.....................................   124

**PART III — PRACTICE MANAGEMENT FOR NURSE
                 PRACTITIONERS**   127

Chapter 10 — Private Practice as a Business   129

    Self-Proprietorship............................   129
    Private Practice as a Profit-Making Business......   132
    Summary.....................................   141

Preface

Nursing in America today is an essential component of our entire health care delivery system. Without nursing, clients and health care delivery personnel would be unable to complement one another for delivery of prevention and healing techniques. One major reason for this fact is that nurses are America's single largest body of health care delivery personnel. Another important reason is that nurses offer the public a huge resource of professional expertise for prevention and treatment of disease.

Techniques of health care delivery range from those in the most complex of hospitals to those in simple clinics in isolated parts of America, from the physician, generally a spearhead for providing care, to the nurse's aide. Nurses represent a large number of personnel between the physician and client and are found throughout the country. All health facilities and personnel accept the dentist, physician, and physical therapist as providers via two mechanisms: the eight-hour shift, employed by an institution, and the self-employed providers offering their care on a fee-for-service or fee-for-treatment basis. Why have nurses avoided the unique mechanism of fee-for-service in caring for people?

Nurses can be self-employed as general practitioners, offering a wide range of professional skills, or as specialists, offering a specialized area of skills. Nurses practice skillfully but are employed by an institution, for a yearly salary. They have not seen their way out of the institution to being self-employed and billing clients on a fee-for-service basis.

The profession needs to develop this modality as a new way to practice nursing if it is to upgrade health care delivery in America. Nursing must become a change agent for the betterment of the field itself and for the health of the public it serves.

This work will explore methods and procedures for developing and managing your own "nursing practice." I coined the term "nursing office" after opening my office, the first in New York State, in 1971, thus setting a precedent. This office, where nurses provide care or practice nursing, is much like

ix

a physician's office, except that the physician practices medicine and nurses practice nursing. Clients and nurses seemed to respond more favorably to the term "nursing practice," as they could comprehend the nurses' role more clearly with it.

Although being self-employed is not for every nurse, all should be familiar with how to develop and manage a nursing practice. Then they can decide if this new approach is for them or not. The concept is a challenge and offers something new, different, and yet extremely professional to the nurses of today, something they have been requesting. Nurses working for themselves must use sound judgment and be competent practitioners to provide nursing out of the hospital, in a client's home, or in their own private offices.

I do not want anyone to think that this idea is designed to compete against physicians and their private practices, hospitals, clinics, nursing homes, or any other current outlets for health care delivery. The concept offered here is designed only to be an adjunct to current sources of health care and to give nurses a position of real professional responsibility. Nurses can work in their traditional places of employment and practice from their offices or just practice nursing from their offices.

This text will relate the history of my practice, revealing experiences that are invaluable; it is a tool for organizing and managing your practice, as an individual or in groups. You may find it helpful to keep this book in your personal library and refer to it, even if you decide private practice is not for you. Remember, not all nurses will care to work this way, just as not all physicians do. The difference is that all physicians have information available to them on practicing through an office and nurses have not until now. This material may help you to make a meaningful decision about your professional future.

Nursing educators will probably find that this book can help to stimulate their students, the future practitioners of our profession. It is in education that this concept should have begun. This book is for student nurses and nurses at many levels of practice. It is not necessarily for those nurses already managing their own private practice. Nurses represent a gigantic number of personnel, who are able to make a meaningful impact in their profession. A proactive change in the nursing profession on a broad scale is due, as there never has been one before.

Support from nurses, physicians, and health care institutions will strengthen this new and exciting mode of practice for the mutual benefit of consumers and health care personnel. I feel strongly that if even a small percentage of nurses in this country opened private practices, there would be enough public support to allow this system to flourish.

Acknowledgments

Special thanks and gratitude go to Barbara Schwarz, B.A., M.L.S. She continually gave her unrelenting aid and much of her time in assisting with the preparation of this text. Her knowledge of librarianship was invaluable.
Esther Stiles, B.S., M.Ed., CPS, also provided a great deal of her time. Much gratitude goes to her as well for her secretarial assistance.
The support offered me through the implementation of my nursing practice by three excellent nurses and friends, Marilyn, Flo, and John, merits special recognition and appreciation.

Part I

Introduction to Private Practice

Chapter 1

Why Private Practice?

ABOUT PRIVATE PRACTICE

As New York State's first private nurse practitioner, I shall try to explain how you can manage your own office. This can be a true challenge for you, a member of the nursing profession.

The nursing practice is an office staffed by a nurse who provides nursing care. This care is not free for your clients; they pay you on a fee-for-service basis, just as they do physicians when they visit their offices. This book will explain the historical events of my practice up to the present. My experience will help you understand more clearly how to manage your own practice.

The concept of the nursing office, or nursing practice as it will be called from here on, is not a tradition in registered nursing practice. Nurses usually work in institutions for a yearly salary. However, nurses can move into the private sector, as many have, and find it extremely rewarding. You may wonder why you have not entered private practice before!

Abdellah says that as nurse practitioners become recognized and accepted for their long-needed contributions to health care, there will be hope of achieving improved health care for all Americans.[1]

Potentially, all nursing services are available in the nursing practice. You decide those that are not offered. How to make this professional judgment is discussed in a later chapter. You may begin to sense the real responsibility and creativity that you can enjoy with private practice.

Following chapters explain and further develop the concept of the nursing practice. This text is for your continued use since it discusses how to conduct a business that provides nursing care to the public through your own institution. Nurses, each and every one, are institutions unto themselves. Your institution may be your nursing practice.

Responsibilities To Recognize

It is necessary to strongly emphasize that any time nurses practice nursing, they must be cognizant of the rules and regulations governing their practice in their locale. This applies whether the nurses are practicing in private practices, separate from the physician by geographical distances, or in hospitals where physicians are geographically close.

In either situation, the nurse must know when he or she needs to obtain a physician's order before providing care. Sometimes a physician's order is not needed before a nurse practices nursing; more often than not, though, an order from a physician is needed, whether you practice in an urban, rural, or suburban area.

Two important factors must be remembered regarding delivery of nursing care from a nursing practice. First, the nurse must practice nursing in a professional and legal manner as mandated by the locale. Second, in order for the business to flourish, the nurse must practice sound business techniques.

Purpose of the Office

Nurses delivering care through their nursing practices are an extension of current nursing service. Nurses practicing this way will be able to meet clients who ordinarily would not go to a physician or hospital. Also, with the growth of nursing practices, more clients could be discharged from hospitals earlier. The nurse in private practice would provide in-office or home-visit care.

Brickner et al. explain that contemporary health care is designed with the expectation that sick people go to hospitals for health care. Many people cannot or do not use this established health care system. The unreached groups are the derelict and homeless, homebound sick people, and the aged who have borderline physical capacity and may not need hospitalization.[2]

The concept of private practice deals with direct client care by nurses and their collaboration with and referral by physicians. (Later, this will be expanded in great detail so that your practice may be an active one.)

One magnanimous aspect of nursing practice as well as of the nursing profession is the fact that nurses are teachers. As a nurse delivering care to your clients from your practice, you will be able to teach them a great deal about prevention and treatment. This alone will help to curtail health care costs to the public.

Kinlein says that to assess and deliver the nursing needs of the public, the setting has to be changed to contact those in need of nursing care.[3]

Helen Kitchen Branson, R.N., M.A., in her article, "A New Nurse for the New Health Care," in *Nursing Care,* September 1977, page 29, explains what Renilda Hilkemeyer, R.N., Director of Nursing at the Anderson Hospital and

Tumor Institute in Houston, Texas, said in a recent address to medical personnel. Hilkemeyer feels that nurses should expand their roles. Added roles could include giving physical examinations, Pap smears, and pelvic examinations; reading coronary-care monitors; and regulating medications. Nurses should relieve physicians of some medical care, leading to better client care.

As a nurse with a private practice, you will have an opportunity to take on some overlapping physician roles where appropriate while treating and caring for your clients. This is part of the purpose of a nursing practice—to more fully treat your clients; to develop collaboration with physicians; and to enhance your skills, capabilities, and teaching.

PRACTICING NURSING IN A MODERN SOCIETY

Mauksch says the emergence of the *nurse practitioner* may be a most significant event in nursing. This role is unique and will have an impact on health care. Due to its uniqueness it may become nursing's means of survival and an answer to society's search for better, more comprehensive health, illness, and preventative care.

To understand the significance of this role and the nature of the nursing care it provides and to justify speculating about it, it must be examined within the context of the changing society that it serves.[4]

One of the problems of nursing in modern society is the attitude of the nurses themselves. Many seem to be reluctant to generate betterment for themselves, their profession, or their clients. A lackadaisical air seems to prevail among many nurses to let the current system of nursing go along as it is.

Many problems seem to stem from nurses themselves, says Fromm. Widespread lack of awareness among nurses of the need to organize and to advance the nursing profession so that it really is professional is a huge problem.[5]

Nurses should become more cognizant of society's needs and their profession's needs and upgrade nursing so that it could better serve more people. The move by nurses into the nursing practice arena of health care delivery will do just that.

Reviewing the American health care system shows emerging roles and specialties with many unmet needs. The nurse practitioner is one such role, which is being developed and refined. It is beginning to fill critical gaps in health care, says Alexander.[6]

The Client Would Benefit

Everyone coming into contact with the nurse in private practice can benefit. The clients would be the first to receive immediate and direct benefits, as their access to a huge group of professional health care delivery (HCD) personnel would be increased. Clients could stay out of the hospital and at home with loved ones and family members more often because the private practitioner could make a home visit to provide adequate, professional care. Hospitals are overcrowded; this would tend to reduce this problem. The private practitioner's fee for care to the client would be lower than that of a hospital. The types of nursing care that could be provided appear in Chapter 4.

The client receiving nursing care at home from the nurse in private practice also reaps the benefit of one-to-one nursing and more of the nurse's time. Increased time enhances communication with the client and allows for teaching the client about his or her care.

The discharged client may visit the nurse's office for follow-up care also. Whether a home visit or office visit occurs depends upon the client's situation. Making yourself known to your community will enhance your client load, because care will be requested by clients once they know you exist.

A client who ordinarily visits an emergency department (ED) every month for vitamin B_{12} injections for pernicious anemia may receive them at home or at a local nursing practice. If a client visits the ED for any care on a routine outpatient basis and has to come to that ED via ambulance, the ED nurse could refer the client to a local nursing practice. The nurse in private practice could make a home visit, saving the client the expense and hardship of the ambulance ride.

The Physician Would Benefit

Hospital physicians would benefit since they would no longer be forced to practice nursing as they so often are when the roles of each profession overlap. There are not enough staff nurses in the hospitals; thus, physicians are often busy performing care that nurses could provide. Discharging patients from a hospital to a nursing practice for home care is an excellent way to provide quality, professional care and reduce the role of the overtaxed physician.

When the institution nurse or physician discharges a client to a local nursing practice for follow-up care, they would have to consult by phone or in person with the staff of the nursing practice to ensure continuity of professional care.

Physicians outside the hospital setting could take advantage of a nursing practice by referring clients to that practice for quality care.

The Hospital Would Benefit

Hospital staffs often complain of overcrowding; they cannot admit as many clients every day as they would like. If staffs were to refer some of them to nursing practices, this problem would be greatly reduced.

Physicians could often refer clients to a nursing practice rather than admit them to a hospital. Letters of introduction to physicians and health care agencies and consultations with them provide the trust and confidence that encourage referrals to your practice.

The Emergency Department Would Benefit

Local EDs would benefit because they are often overcrowded with routine clients who come to them every week, every two weeks, or every month for ongoing nursing care. Often, the client needing a catheter change biweekly as a standard part of care repeatedly visits the ED for this. This service takes the busy ED nurse away from his or her true role: caring for clients requiring specialized, expert emergency nursing.

ED overcrowding could be eased. And, the client who needs ongoing care could obtain more nursing time at a lower cost from a nurse in private practice. Therefore, ED nurses should refer ongoing care clients to a local nursing practice.

Removing Threats

When opening your practice, be certain to visit EDs, hospitals, and physicians so that they will know about your practice, and so that they will not feel threatened. EDs, hospitals, and physicians can be easily threatened because they may believe you are taking business away from them. Reinforce that your practice is to be an adjunct to the care provided by them. Hopefully, they will begin referring clients to you.

This example shows why the in-service education departments of institutions should teach courses to their staffs about private practice by nurses. Any threat of a nursing practice has to be erased, since it is a valuable method of health care.

My experience showed that the nurses themselves were the most threatened by this concept. They believed it was illegal to practice this way and thought I wanted *all* of their clients and all of the physicians' clients, too. Neither was true. These threatened feelings have been gone for years now. Referrals come in from ED nurses, physicians, hospitals, druggists, supply houses, other professionals, lay people, and all sorts of other places.

The Insurance Company Would Benefit as a Private Insurer

Insurance companies that pay providers for HCD would benefit. Their cash payments to physicians and institutions would decrease, because they could pay nurse practitioners for similar services at a lower, and yet meaningful, rate.

The insurance company would retain much revenue through lowered costs of claims. Then it could pass this savings on to clients who purchase health insurance. Premiums for insurance policies could be reduced. The insurance companies could contract with nurse practitioners for life insurance physicals. The nurse's fee would be less than a physician's for the physical exam.

Insurance companies are private insurers because the public can purchase their health care insurance privately. Examples are Blue Cross, Blue Shield, Major Medical, and any other private insurance company. Presently, nurses or nurse practitioners are not covered in private health insurance programs on a fee-for-service basis. However, clients are willing to visit the nursing practice even though they pay personally. They do so because the nurses there provide more time with the clients. The nurse in private practice teaches, offers emotional support, will make home visits when needed, provides many of the same services as a physician, and often charges less than a physician. It is not that physicians never provide these services, but nurses are more available to provide them than physicians. Thus, in-depth collaboration should be established between physicians and nurses to promote the concept of private nursing practice.

The Federal Government Would Benefit as a Public Insurer

The federally funded programs to provide health care insurance could benefit tremendously if nurses entered private practice on a large scale. These federal health care insurance providers are Medicare, Medicaid, and National Health Insurance. They are funded by tax dollars from the public, and they have such large payments to HCD providers that they are running out of money. By reducing HCD costs by paying nurses in private practices, the government would save a great deal of money now paid out to other providers. The new providers would be nurses in nursing practices.

On December 13, 1977, a bill was signed into law (P.L. 95–210) extending Medicare and Medicaid reimbursement for nurse practitioners' services in rural health clinics. This law is an excellent beginning for fee-for-service payment for nursing care, but it is restrictive to the nursing practice concept in two ways. First, the nursing practice is not a clinic, and, second, the constraining effect of this law is apparent in that payment for nursing care is limited to rural areas. The concept of nursing practice is viable in rural as well as all other locales. Hopefully, Congress will extend this coverage to broader geographical settings, since the health needs of the public are just as demanding and pressing in all settings.

The American public would benefit in that eventually the taxes needed to support public insurance could be reduced or at least not increased.

Also, America is a role model for many other countries. If it were demonstrated that a tax savings could be passed on to the public at the same time the public was obtaining quality health care closer to home, more easily, more cheaply, and in larger quantity, other countries might adopt this plan. If this concept is well accepted in Washington, D.C., the government might provide federal money to assist nurses in getting their practices started.

Unions with Health Care Funds Would Benefit

Any union, large or small, local or national, could save union and member funds by encouraging members to visit nursing practices more frequently. The savings to the member would stem from the reduced premiums for health care insurance that union members pay.

These members represent a large section of society, and their support of nursing practices would be valuable. So many of these members go to physicians, hospitals, or EDs for routine, continuous care—the kind of care a competent nurse can easily provide from a nursing practice.

Benefits to the Registered Nurse Would Be Endless

This section may make you feel that the primary reason for creating nursing practices is to benefit nurses. Perhaps a majority of the benefits would go to nurses; however, these benefits are passed on directly to the public, physicians, institutions, the government, and clients.

Agree asks why nurses venture into independent practice: many report deep frustration at not being able to practice the full scope of nursing in an emotionally satisfying environment. Nurses seem determined to achieve greater professional and personal fulfillment. All are not economically motivated; however, financial considerations are a factor.[7]

Nurses entering private practice would find fulfillment in their new roles. They could spend more time with clients, on a more desirable one-to-one basis. With this time, nurses could provide a great service to clients—teaching them about their (the clients') bodies and their health care. Finally, nurses would realize much job satisfaction and feel and see their clients benefit by this new role.

Nurses would be able to practice their skills in a fashion becoming to them. So many positive results would occur from nurses developing nursing practices that it almost compels them to enter this role.

Alexander reassures that the nurse practitioner role has the potential to enliven the nursing profession. This role offers a new means for professional growth, upward mobility, higher income, and satisfaction and recognition.[8]

PUBLIC IMAGE OF NURSING WOULD CHANGE

There is a dichotomy in nursing today. The nurse is a person as well as a professional. Which image fits the nurse? Nurses' images and expectations of the profession have greatly changed. The public has a false concept of nursing, and it influences them to enter the profession.

Lyons states that nursing is considered a worthwhile job. It demands a certain personality. The nurse is usually portrayed as practical, competent, broadminded, and dedicated. This portrayal is tinted in a way, leading others to believe that there are rewards for the suffering that nurses experience.

This image is of the general nurse, while psychiatric nursing is thought unworthy by the parents of those considering nursing school.

This is a popular concept, responsible for the fact that a decision to enter nursing is often made before the candidate has a realistic idea of what nursing is.[9]

So the dichotomy remains between the public image and the professional image, which is one of a highly skilled, interdependent professional who realizes he or she cannot be all things to all people. Nurses should keep their relationships with their clients on a professional level. But the public does not see the nurse as a person, only as a professional who is consistently described by the same public image.

This dichotomy frustrates students, because once they are involved with nursing schools they find it difficult to cope with the extensive skill and knowledge that they are expected to learn and retain. The public realizes nurses are professional but fails to realize to what extent.

One reason that nurses have not entered private practice is because the educational system has been service oriented. Students learn nursing through apprenticeship in the hospital as a clinical agency; they also learn to remain in that authoritarian regime with rigid adherence to routine.

As nursing becomes more educationally oriented and nurses begin to demonstrate to themselves, other professionals, and the public that they have something of value to offer and then offer it through their own offices, the public will adopt a new image of the profession. Nurses themselves can take a new pride in being more complete health care providers with the importance of practicing through nursing offices.

The public will have much more contact with nursing and demand to utilize its skills more than ever. The public image of nursing will be changed to the level where it should be.

Schlotfeldt says nurses will capitalize on politicians' interest in providing services to the elderly and to those needing sustained care over long time periods. Nurses will establish nursing as a profession whose members are responsible and willing to be held accountable for their health care. Nurses will ensure that they are recognized for being competent practitioners, and that they will collaborate with other professionals in planning and carrying out needed health care. Nurses should take every opportunity in planning for their future.[10]

Role Clarity

When roles are ambiguous, anxiety and tension increase. This pressure arises from roles being defined differently from institution to institution where nurses are employed and educated as well as from their states' definitions.

Nurses have an image of their role and can perform well if given the freedom to work within their state's definition. They could practice nursing through their own office following their state's definition and setting policy for their private practice.

Much job tension is created by institutions demanding that nurses take on heavier patient loads (which is unsafe and lowers the quality of care provided). Also, limitations are placed on nurses regarding what they can and cannot do. Thus, their need for role clarity increases, as does tension, while satisfaction and performance go down.

Role ambiguity leads to less productivity and increased defensiveness. Nurses escape role ambiguity tension by withdrawing and doing as employers say. This phenomenon is common in today's hospitals, and investigators described the nursing profession as having a blurred image due to this ambiguity. Recent technical, medical, and social changes have resulted in unclear demands and definitions for nursing, claims Lyons.[11] By accepting traditional roles too easily, nurses may be perpetuating an outdated and confusing role for themselves.

The new and challenging role of being self-employed as a private practitioner can be the answer to role ambiguity found in institutions today. Nurses could practice under one definition of nursing—their state's—rather than each institution's definition. This would reduce tension and increase job satisfaction and performance.

Nurses are in the middle between the physician and the hospital structure. They either cope with it or leave. You shouldn't leave your job hastily; it is extremely important as both a source of income and a worthy place for practicing nursing. A challenging goal would be one where 10–15 percent of America's nurses enter private practices within the next few years.

As a profession, we need more public and mass media exposure to change the public and peer group image, as well as to clear up our roles as nurses.

Many states in America are rewriting their laws to encourage nurses to clarify and redesign their role.

Table 1-1 Force Field Analysis—Why Private Practice?

Should nurses enter private practice on a large scale?

Forces Towards Private Practice	Forces Against Private Practice
1. People need greater access to health care delivery. • Nursing practices will create greater accessibility to nursing care. • A huge body of untapped nursing ability would be utilized. • Communities would benefit from nursing practices.	1. Suspicion exists that the American Medical Association does not want nurses to practice in this manner. The *assumed* reason is that this model of practice is reserved, and only legal, for physicians. Assumptions hold nursing from progress.
2. Nurses practice preventative care.	2. Nurses are reluctant to make any change.
3. Nursing is a profession, and professions are in a constant state of change.	3. Nurses do not want changes in general. Older nurses in high positions, nursing's role models, are reluctant to change.
4. Nurses could spend more time with their clients.	4. Nurses do not want increased responsibility and are reluctant to change their comfortable, current roles.
5. It unifies nurses, increases their communication and strength.	5. It is difficult to change people's attitudes. Nurses are unable to coexist with each other due to their inability to come to terms with each other.
6. Many nurses want this change.	6. Peer group support is lacking.
7. When the concept of nursing practice becomes widespread, banks will probably provide funding to beginning nurse practitioners.	7. Start-up costs are difficult to meet. Nurses are reluctant to provide start-up costs through personal or bank financing.
8. Nurses may have realized the need for it while studying nursing.	8. Private practice has not been offered in nursing school curricula.
9. It allows for more autonomy of the nurse.	9. Some nurses do not want autonomy.
10. It is rewarding and satisfying.	10.
11. A wide variety of nursing services are available.	11.
12. Nurses can make house calls when physicians cannot.	12.
13. There are few restrictions as to geographic location.	13.
14. A nursing practice can be established in a variety of settings: your home, a store front, a professional building, etc.	14. Not all nurses will be willing to expend the effort needed to develop a private practice.
15. State laws governing nursing usually allow private practice.	15. Nurses believe too many assumptions about private practice; they rarely seek validation.

Forces Towards Private Practice	Forces Against Private Practice
16. It reduces overcrowding in physicians' offices, EDs, and hospitals.	16.
17. It would create jobs for many highly skilled and unemployed nurses.	17.
18. It lowers health care costs to the public.	18. Many nurses assume that the American Medical Association has kept nurses from being quoted in fee schedules for third-party payment on a fee-for-service basis.
19. It could reduce insurance premiums of private insurance companies.	19. Private insurance companies have failed to include nurses in fee schedules on a fee-for-service basis.
20. The majority of clients are willing to pay personally for nursing service from a private practice. This is in view of the fact that insurance companies exclude nurses from fee schedules, on a fee-for-service basis for third-party payment.	20.
21. It reduces taxes needed to fund public insurance programs.	21.
22. It creates closer relationships with physicians to benefit HCD.	22. Nurses more than physicians are reluctant to develop a closer relationship. This prohibits collaboration for the betterment of HCD.
23. It reduces transportation costs for clients as nurses could visit clients at home, several times a day or week, as needed, in the form of community rounds.	23.
24. Utilizing nurses in this manner will alleviate the physician shortage.	24.
25. The nursing profession would become a leader in HCD.	25.
26. Nurses in or out of private practice would achieve greater self-awareness, confidence, and assertiveness. They would have a potential for greater collaboration with physicians, acquisition of new skills, and provision of increased time to teach their clients.	26.
27. Nurses could openly demonstrate their professionalism.	27.
28. Union health insurance costs would be reduced through utilization of nursing practices.	28. Nursing needs to increase the awareness of union leaders and others about what nursing can offer health care recipients.

Several factors influence role expansion for nurses: the shortage of primary care physicians, the federal government, the physician's assistant movement, the growing complexity of acute hospital care, educational reform, and the women's liberation movement. Laws governing nursing are changing, actually supporting role expansion, says Bullough.[12]

Escape from Traditional Roles

Hospital employment is thought of as a family where roles are "old shoe." Expectations and performances have become well-meshed, so the nurses can relax in them. The hospital family is a center of role allocation and assumes an important position in solving role strain.

Formal removal from these relationships is difficult, and informal removal arouses individual guilt feelings and pressure from others. For a nurse to leave the hospital as a place of employment can be very difficult. However, if you do and experience the freedom of private practice, you can erase your guilt feelings and realize your potential to nursing. If nurses truly want to practice in a new way, they should be willing to take some personal risks.

Mauksch says it is difficult to take risks. It requires overcoming your initial socialization and timidity. Individuals must decide who they are and what it is they want to do, and then do it.[13]

SUMMARY

The force field analysis, shown in Table 1–1, concisely illustrates positive and negative views regarding private practice. The positive forces indicate the need for growth of the nursing profession toward private practice.

NOTES

1. Faye G. Abdellah, Ph.D., "Nurse Practitioners and Nursing Practice," *American Journal of Public Health* 66, no. 3 (March 1976): 246.

2. Philip W. Brickner et al., "Outreach to Welfare Hotels, the Homebound, the Frail," *American Journal of Nursing* 76, no. 5 (May 1976): 762.

3. M. Lucille Kinlein, "Independent Nurse Practitioner," *Nursing Outlook* 20 (January 1972): 23.

4. Ingeborg G. Mauksch, "Nursing Is Coming of Age Through the Practitioner Movement," *American Journal of Nursing* 75, no. 10 (October 1975): 1835.

5. Linda Fromm, "The Problem in Nursing: Nurses!" *Supervisor Nurse* 8, no. 10 (October 1977): 16.

6. Linda Alexander, Ph.D., "The Nurse Practitioner and Professional Growth," *Nurse Practitioner* 1, no. 6 (July-August 1976): 32.

7. Betty C. Agree, "Beginning an Independent Nursing Practice," *American Journal of Nursing* 76, no. 4 (April 1974): 642.

8. Linda Alexander, Ph.D., "The Nurse Practitioner and Professional Growth," *Nurse Practitioner* 1, no. 6 (July-August 1976): 33.

9. Thomas F. Lyons, "Role Clarity, Need for Clarity, Satisfaction, Tension, and Withdrawal," *Organizational Behavior and Human Performance* 6, no. 1 (January 1971): 99.

10. Rozella Schlotfeldt, R.N., Ph.D., F.A.A.N., "Rozella Schlotfeldt Says," *American Journal of Nursing* 76, no. 1: 105.

11. Thomas F. Lyons, "Role Clarity, Need for Clarity, Satisfaction, Tension, and Withdrawal," *Organizational Behavior and Human Performance* 6, no. 1 (January 1971): 103.

12. Bonnie Bullough, "Influences on Role Expansion," *American Journal of Nursing* 76, no. 9 (September 1976): 1476.

13. Ingeborg G. Mauksch, R.N., "Paradox of Risk Takers," *AORN Journal* 25, no. 7 (June 1977): 1307.

Chapter 2

Formal Education as a Pathway to Private Practice

LEADERSHIP THROUGH FORMAL EDUCATION

Nurses can provide their services from private practices, offering an abundance of skills to the public. The knowledge needed to develop and manage a private practice could come from additional formal education. It could come more easily from the incorporation of courses in existing schools of nursing at the generic or graduate level.

McAtee and Silver explain that a nurse completing an additional formal nurse-practitioner program is competent to provide a broader range of health care services. This nurse can assess health status, assume responsibility for management and follow-up, counsel, teach, refer, and create greater continuity of health care for clients. Within guidelines of governing laws, this nurse can make nursing diagnoses and give more treatments to clients.[1]

Why is it that nurses have avoided practicing their profession privately? Nursing in America is an essential component of our entire health care delivery (HCD) system. Without nurses, other health care delivery personnel would not complement one another for maximum health care delivery, since nurses are America's single largest body of HCD personnel. Nurses could rearrange their position in the current system of HCD to take one of leadership.

Nurses have not concerned themselves with professional administrative and management principles and the type of leadership that connotes followers. Thus nursing continues to be perceived in a nonleadership position by the consumer and others, Cutler states.[2]

Why is it then, since nursing is so important, that it has not made a significant contribution to gearing up a change in the way nurses practice? With many members to offer suggestions, why has nursing let other health professions take a leading role in national changes of HCD?

Fowkes and Hunn say that America's health care needs are changing. America's health resources are subjected to severe stress by population growth.

Increasing life expectancy, expanding technology, and new demands from previously neglected groups add to this stress. Furthermore, the complexity of medical care, which involves huge numbers of people in different roles, presents problems in providing comprehensive health care. It is obvious that our present health care system is not capable of meeting all the needs of the people. The health care system needs change. Innovative uses of the health labor force can be an answer to this.[3]

The Problem

The original and still operant problem is changing the locus of practice for the nurse. This problem is heightened by the rigid attitudes nurses have about where they practice and their strong reluctance to change this locus. Thus, nurses are so secure and so conditioned to practicing in a traditional setting that they are not willing to change behavior or policy.

Nurses need to realize their full potential as health care providers. Then, consumers would fully benefit from nursing care. A role change from passive to aggressive is needed if nursing is to play a major part in creating better health care in America, say Sateren and Westover.[4]

If nurses began to practice nursing from the private sector it would constitute a dynamic change. This concept of the private sector connotes a high level of professionalism. Nurses have greater potential to reach the public when the private sector of nursing practice is added to current sectors. Private practices can be established in rural, suburban, and urban settings.

Lenburg says that nursing can only be recognized as a profession in a knowledge-oriented, not task-oriented, environment. This means that nurses would be expected to utilize the knowledge they have and take the initiative, not waiting for directions from others.[5]

In the private sector nurses will be capable of using their knowledge in a more realistic and meaningful fashion.

Mechanisms for Providing Health Care Delivery

HCD facilities and their personnel accept the dentist, physician, physical therapist, and others as providers of health care via two mechanisms:

1. the eight-hour shift as an employee of a given institution
2. the self-employed provider offering services on a fee-for-service or fee-for-treatment basis in an office, in the patient's home, or through privileges in an institution to visit patients there and bill them directly

Why is it that nurses have decided to exclude themselves from the second mechanism, when it is obvious that it works and meets a great many needs of the public?

The Self-Employed Nurse

Nurses could easily be self-employed as general practitioners, offering a wide range of professional skills, or as specialists, offering a specialized area of nursing skills. They practice this way now, but only through the first mechanism, the eight-hour shift. In this type of practice nurses sell their skills and knowledge to an employing institution for a dollar amount over a year's time. It is difficult for them to see their way *out* of these institutions with the same degree of professionalism that they now have while practicing *in* these institutions.

Nurses are threatened by the concept and reality of private practice. They avoid it or resist seeing its true potential. The arena of private practice has traditionally been regarded as territory held and preserved only for the physician. The need exists for nurses to move into this arena.

Nurses can employ themselves, as they themselves are institutions. They could sell their skills and knowledge to an employing client for a dollar amount over a span of time, say a half hour to an hour, much as existing self-employed providers do. Fee-for-service or fee-for-treatment is a consideration as well as the amount of skill, knowledge, preparation, and responsibility needed to perform the task when accounting for the actual cost to the client.

Simms stated that nurse practitioners could earn adequate incomes in rural or inner city areas. They could also keep health care costs low for their services. Many nurses are prepared to practice in these areas after nursing school. Nursing education *now* provides its graduates with the knowledge and skills to provide much of the health care service that is lacking and could be met by private practice.[6]

Nurses could deliver a great deal of health care through their private practices, aiding the present institutions of HCD in meeting the community's needs. However, nurses seem to be uninterested in this style, even in view of the fact that a great deal of favorable mass media has been available since 1972 supporting private practice. Probably much of this disinterest in private practice is due to the lack of exposure to it from nursing schools throughout the country. The schools of nursing provide their graduates with the necessary knowledge and skills to practice nursing but do not offer knowledge and skills to become entrepreneurs or private practitioners.

Nurses are aware that nursing as a health profession must select the changes that will strengthen it for people rather than the kind that continue to fragment and destroy it, says Alexander. Nurses have been directly available, accessible, and acceptable to all groups, such as physicians, hospital administrators, and the public. These groups endeavored to help control and define the role and function of nurses, when nurses should have done it themselves. In the midst of a health care crisis, nurses have attempted to meet the nursing needs of clients working within a disorganized, fragmented, and obsolete system of management.[7]

Traditional Settings Cloud Innovation

Working in the nurse's traditional setting is expected and taught. It is easily accepted and reinforced by older nurses who have moved up the career ladder to a position of greater authority. They are reluctant to change, thus holding our profession back, prohibiting nurses from delivering additional health care.

Alexander says nurses discount the hidden curriculum within schools of nursing. Here clinical practice occurs in bureaucratic agencies, hospitals, public health departments. In these settings students learn the power structure and the nurse's place in this working framework.[8]

Nurses should develop the modality of private practice for HCD if nursing is to upgrade its delivery of nursing care to the public. Nursing must become a real change agent for better public health care.

To elicit change in the formal organization of the health care system, nurse practitioners need to devise a workable solution. Then they need to have the solution accepted, negotiate it into practice, and develop a public awareness as successful and helpful health care innovators, says Aeschliman.[9]

There are several articles and textbooks on the subject of change. The concepts in this text guide you in actually changing your modality of professional practice from institutional to private. As a side effect of implementing private practices, change will be evoked. Evolving through this change will be a hair-raising process, but it is within most nurses' reach.

A move into private practice should be given careful thought and time. Rushing into it may prove devastating to you and dangerous to your clients.

Gretchen T. Randolph, in her article "Experiences in Private Practice," *Journal of Psychiatric Nursing,* volume 13, November-December 1975, page 16, explains that her decision to enter private practice was not immediate or clear-cut. She evolved into private practice over a period of several years of self-evaluation.

Schorr says that three open forum speakers concluded that to become a private nurse practitioner, nurses need courage, experience, and maturity.[10]

Innovation is also retarded by the nursing education system. The educational process is geared to demonstrate delivery of nursing care in an institution. If nurses learn to practice in a setting away from an institution, such as a clinic, they will probably find that this isolated setting is directly controlled by the parent institution.

Nursing schools teach via apprenticeships. The student receives classroom and laboratory instruction and practices while learning in a hospital affiliated with the nursing school. The educational process affords no mention of or exposure to a nursing private practice. No learning experiences utilize a private practice as a realistic clinical experience, with an instructor of nursing available and a letter of agreement or contract between this new clinical agency, the private practice, and the school of nursing.

Fowkes and Hunn explain that efforts are under way to increase numbers of health personnel. These efforts do not provide the complete solution. Perhaps the best solution to the increasing demands for health services involves the greater use of existing personnel resources. A logical approach is to delegate certain aspects of medical care traditionally provided by the physician to new types of health professionals. This would increase the quantity of services available. If nurses moved into the primary care system, they could assume more significant role responsibilities. This would meet the needs of the nursing profession as well as the demands of the health care system.[11]

Reform is needed so that the public can obtain easy, direct access to nursing care at several locations throughout the community. Nursing schools need to incorporate courses teaching the concept of private practice as an adjunct to traditional teaching methods. This would enable future graduates to decide if private practice is realistic for them and, if it is, to be competent managers and deliverers of nursing care at the same time.

Safety, Responsibility, and Experience

A few years of actual nursing practice are safest before a nurse attempts to enter private practice. In order to work as a graduate nurse in most states the graduate from a nursing school usually has to be employed by an institution with 50 beds or more. This ensures safety and quality control since a head nurse and supervisor are available for immediate consultation and assistance. Once taught the managerial skills, and after some experience, the graduate could enter private practice. Perhaps laws could be changed to allow new graduates to be employed by private practitioners with 50 or more clients.

Private practice will not appeal to all nurses, just as psychiatric nursing and medical-surgical nursing are unappealing to some. If a meaningful percentage of nurses entered the realm of private practice, the public could more easily receive health care at a lower cost. Nurses in private practice can provide services traditionally available as well as those overlapping with physicians' care. The physician generally receives more financial reimbursement for the same nursing type service than a nurse does. The nurse can offer more time to the client to teach, outline and provide care, and answer questions. Nurses would be practicing their profession in a more realistic manner.

Nurses considering this modality of practice are strongly advised to acquire some meaningful experience in a typical HCD setting. They should decide if they are personally responsible enough to practice from a private setting where they will have to rely on their own judgment and knowledge more than they will in an institutional setting. A nurse who realizes that he or she will not be safe in private practice and so does not enter it, is safe and professional. They should continue working in a setting they feel is comfortable.

Rosamond Gabrielson, president of the American Nurses Association (ANA), told National Student Nurses Association members the ANA Board of Directors confirms that graduates of diploma schools of nursing provide the greatest amount of professional nursing care in America. Many of them fill critical leadership positions; they are qualified through experience, self-development, and continuing education. The ANA board recommended that every program unit in ANA consider the special needs and interests of diploma school graduates when developing their plans for each biennium. The Commission on Nursing Education should identify means for diploma school graduates to continue their education. The Commission on Economic and General Welfare should explore ways to allow for horizontal and vertical mobility. Recognition of an individual's experience, competency, and demonstrated abilities is needed, says Schorr.[12]

The tremendous amount of clinical experience diploma school students receive qualifies them as the most likely to move quickly into private practice. However, a nurse from any level of education is able to do so by law. Just because the law allows all nurses in general to enter this practice system doesn't mean that all of them should. You must have insight into your capabilities and only enter private practice if you feel you are ready.

NURSING EDUCATION

Instructors who could implement a curriculum with lectures about private practice in their syllabus are threatened and reluctant to change because they are unfortunate victims or by-products of the clinical settings where nursing has been taught traditionally. This system needs internal revamping to meet public demands on health providers. Nurses may feel this demand acutely because they come in contact with a great number of clients daily for a lengthy period of time. During this time clients communicate their needs to the nurses.

Haase states that each nurse at any level of practice should have a sense of dignity. Differences among practitioners need to be institutionalized into a role structure. This would enable the public to identify nurse behavior. This can be achieved by title, by setting of practice, or by position in a hierarchical or collegial organizational structure.

Nursing suffers from a lack of personnel that are prepared academically and clinically to teach, to practice competently at more sophisticated levels, to administer, to research, and to negotiate with other health care systems that put pressure on nursing. Nurses lack a voice in top-level policy decisions concerning the direction of health care. Their lack of credentials may encourage this omission. Often articles and viewpoints about the future of health care are derived from magazines for physicians, administrators, and economists. Few nurses write about their own valid and realistic views and roles.[13]

The issues presented here are major forces that retard the huge challenge of curriculum reform in nursing. Nurses must take an active role in changing nursing so that it meets their needs as well as the needs of the public.

To summarize, Jones and Jones say that the nursing instructor is perceived by the student as the most influential person in nursing. Since nurses are educated in different levels of nursing programs, this could be a reason they define their roles differently.[14]

Perhaps change could be introduced through longer programs of education, as graduates from longer programs seem to be more professionally oriented. The influential nursing instructors could easily begin lecturing about the concept of private practice.

Judith L. Sateren and Devra E. Westover, in their article, "Baccalaureate Preparation for Action-Practice Nursing," in *Nurse Educator,* volume no. 5, September-October 1978, page 12, discuss the outcome of two of their projects which took their senior nursing majors into the community for clinical experience in a wide range of ambulatory health care settings.

They employed a one-month interim of intensive study to build upon the students' knowledge base, thus using their enriched knowledge base to refine nursing skills. Higher level nursing diagnosis, decisions, and judgments were encouraged.

The health care settings used for clinical experience were public schools, private and public health clinics, physicians' offices, private and county hospital nurseries, and well-child clinics in inner-city, suburban, and rural areas. Community mental health centers throughout the state provided added clinical settings.

The students worked closely with the nurse practitioners and the other members of the health team, observing nurses practicing in expanded roles.

The goals of this curriculum change included emphasizing health promotion and maintenance and provision of a broad range of community-based facilities for clinical experience. Also provided was a wide range of learning experiences as well as opportunities to practice expanded skills. Experiences to foster creative, independent, and responsible learning were provided. Significant changes in the curriculum were undertaken.

Overall, the outcomes of this project were positive. Most striking was the fact that students demonstrated a higher level of independent decision making and a greater sense of accountability.

One student refined her independent decision-making skills by providing physical and developmental assessments and vision, nutrition, and hearing tests for children.

This experience taught students the importance of planning and providing health care with the client. Much of the students' prior experience with clients was in the institutional setting. Bureaucratic red tape at times determined clients' needs. They were limited often in their health care activities by rigid hospital routines and by the medical-model approach to health care. The students in the project based nursing decisions on professional knowledge and health team goals.

The authors felt that the results of the project were valuable enough for all of the students in the nursing school. Plans were made to include components of the project in the general curriculum.

Hopefully, other schools of nursing will become progressive and begin to make changes in their curriculums. Once this trend started, the "domino effect" could bring private practice into full blossom.

Most likely the quality of nursing leadership in the future will be an important factor when determining where the nursing profession is headed. Experimentation with new methods of nursing care delivery is needed. Emphasis on patient-centered care is expected, says Ellis.[15]

Teaching Private Practice

Change is difficult to implement. It can be very difficult and threatening to nurses, nursing students, and nurse instructors. Nursing's major change needs to be in the area of its delivery of public health. The role of the nurse as a private practitioner should be taught at the generic level of nursing education. Instruction can be provided through curriculum by addition of a nursing practice as a clinical setting and as a portion of formal classroom lecture. Teaching this role to those already practicing nursing can be easily implemented through mass media, self-study, or continuing education. It can also be taught as a required core course in nursing programs that offer bachelor's or master's degrees to practicing nurses working toward these degrees.

Elsie Simms in her article, "Preparation for Independent Practice," in *Nursing Outlook,* volume 25, no. 2, February 1977, points out that in 1973, Brown stated that, "Extensive current planning for future health services indicates that to an appreciably greater degree such services will be provided on an ambulatory and at home basis, with greatly increased attention to health maintenance." Thus, nursing educators and students may be considering courses to prepare nurses for the responsibility of private practice.

The public needs education about private practice also. The public will probably be quick to adapt to this because it will be convenient, less costly, and easily accessible to them. It should satisfy the public's needs.

Assumptions About Private Practice

There are other reasons why nurses have not established private practices: the great number of assumptions nurses and student nurses have as to what is required to become a nurse practitioner. The term *nurse* here includes nurse instructors and nurse administrators.

These assumptions and the realities are described in Table 2-1.

The fact is: basically none of these assumptions are true. They are unfounded on fact. To practice nursing is to be a nurse practitioner, and a nurse practitioner can practice privately. Every nurse planning to enter private practice is advised to investigate the rules and regulations governing nursing in his or her locale; generally, nurses may work from private practices.

Curriculum Changes

Tables 2-2 to 2-5 show current curriculums in various level nursing schools. All of the tables omit a section on private practice. If some nursing schools began to offer this study to their students, our profession would soon face a fantastic overhauling.

Simms says research shows that students and faculties in nursing schools prefer courses that would help nurses become entrepreneurs in the practice of nursing.[16]

Clearly, the fourth semester of a typical two-year school of nursing leaves room for a course structured to introduce students to the concept of private practice or to teach the concept itself. Such a course would easily be absorbed into the fourth semester in the elective area or in the Nursing Leadership course. The time has come for our nursing instructors to introduce this concept to their students, so they can decide for themselves if they want private practices. Nursing leaders and instructors who do not at least introduce this concept are being unfair to their students, their profession, and the public. In other words, nursing instructors should not decide to exclude this concept altogether from their curriculum. They should be pleased to have a brave new concept to offer their students since modern society is ready for it. Nurses are

Table 2-1 Assumptions Regarding Development of a Private Practice

Assumptions	Realities
1. A master's degree in nursing is needed.	1. A master's degree is not needed. Generally, you only need be an RN to open a private practice, although a master's degree may aid you in the management of your practice.
2. A bachelor's degree in nursing is needed.	2. A bachelor's degree is not needed. Generally, you only need be an RN to open a private practice, although a bachelor's degree may assist you in the business and management of your practice.
3. A special course preparing you is needed.	3. Generally, there are no regulations requiring a special course as a prerequisite to opening your private practice. Successful completion of a course in private practice may raise your level of competency.
4. Many years of experience as a nurse are needed.	4. Any self-disciplined and resourceful, currently registered nurse may be capable of developing a private practice. A few years of traditional nursing experience would be valuable.
5. A special license is needed.	5. Your current RN license should be sufficient to practice privately.
6. A special exam is needed.	6. Becoming a registered nurse is enough of a challenge and an exam in itself. This should be sufficient to practice privately.
7. A special clearance is needed in the state capital's regulatory agency for nursing.	7. No special clearance is needed. Your state's regulatory agency may be primarily concerned as to whether you have completed nursing school and the state board exams. These comprise your primary clearance as well as a current license to practice registered professional nursing in the state where you practice. They may investigate to verify that you are practicing within the scope of nursing.
8. A special clearance is needed from your state's nursing association.	8. No special clearance is needed. Your state nursing association may be concerned primarily with whether you are a bona fide nursing school graduate and currently licensed practitioner. They may investigate to determine if you are practicing legally.
9. A special clearance or permit or license is needed from the American Nurses Association.	9. The American Nurses Association is not involved with clearances, permits, or licensure. These are the realm of your state's laws.

Assumptions	Realities
10. Only a three-year graduate or higher can practice this way.	10. A registered nurse from any level of education can provide nursing care from a private practice. However, the more clinical experience one has, either from generic education or job experience, the safer the nurse will be in private practice.
11. A two-year graduate cannot open a private practice.	11. An RN from any level of education is potentially capable of private practice. A two-year graduate with a license to practice nursing may practice this way, but some experience would be beneficial.
12. It is illegal to practice this way at all, no matter what the credentials of the nurse are.	12. Generally, for any RN to deliver nursing care from a private practice is legal. The assumption that it is not is without merit.

ready, also; it is the nurses' responsibility to implement private practice.

At any level of generic nursing education, one of the clinical settings for medicine, surgery, pediatrics, obstetrics, psychiatrics, or specialties could be a private nursing practice. This is one of the best ways to introduce the experience of practicing outside a hospital setting. If this study will not fit into an early stage in a given program, it would definitely belong near the program's end, as the students become more sophisticated.

The curricular outline in Table 2-3 of the three-year nursing school shows the most appropriate time to offer a course on private practice would be in the senior year. The spring semester is best because a course on private practice would fit neatly into the sections entitled Nursing Leadership and Senior Nursing.

Table 2-2 Typical Curriculum of a Two-Year Nursing School

Nursing Program

First Semester	English II
Fundamentals of Nursing	*Third Semester*
Anatomy and Physiology	Medical-Surgical Nursing
English I	Microbiology
Psychology I	Speech
Physical Education	Sociology I
Second Semester	*Fourth Semester*
Pediatrics	Psychiatric Nursing
Obstetrical Nursing	Sociology II
Biochemistry	Nursing Leadership
Psychology II	Elective

Table 2-3 Typical Curriculum of a Three-Year Diploma Nursing School

Nursing Program

FRESHMAN YEAR	JUNIOR YEAR
Fall Semester	*Fall Semester*
Fundamentals of Nursing I	Medical-Surgical Nursing I
English I	Sociology I
Psychology I	Microbiology
Inorganic Chemistry	*Spring Semester*
Anatomy	Medical-Surgical Nursing II
Spring Semester	Sociology II
Fundamentals of Nursing II	*Summer Semester*
Organic Chemistry	Psychiatric Nursing
Psychology II	SENIOR YEAR
Physiology	*Fall Semester*
English II	Pediatric Nursing
Summer Semester	Obstetrical Nursing
Fundamentals of Nursing	*Spring Semester*
or	Nursing Leadership
Vacation	Senior Nursing

The three-year diploma school graduate is a strong graduate ready to work in a wide variety of employment situations. All nurse graduates must work in a large institution with over 50 beds while waiting to take their state board exams for nursing. Once these exams are successfully completed, these nurses could quickly enter into private practice. It is recommended, though, that nurses entering private practice have significant experience in a conventional HCD setting. Private nursing practices could soon be conventional HCD settings.

The baccalaureate nursing program is producing a graduate with more overall college preparation. There is a greater amount of time at this level to introduce a course about private nursing practice. As demonstrated in Table 2-4, a good way to introduce such a course of study would be in the Junior year, Semester II, under Systems of Health Care. Also, in the Senior year, Semester I, Community Nursing or Strategies for Change would suit this topic well. Perhaps some of these four-year schools of nursing could even name their course Private Practice. Also, in the Senior year, Semester II, the Nursing Leadership and Nursing Elective slots provide an excellent opportunity for the nursing school to teach a course on private practice.

Table 2-4 Typical Curriculum of a Baccalaureate Nursing Program

Nursing Program

FRESHMAN YEAR	Human Development
Semester I	Elective
Inorganic Chemistry	JUNIOR YEAR
Anatomy and Physiology I	*Semester I*
Sociology I	Fundamentals of Nursing
Psychology I	Nursing Methodology
English I	Speech
Semester II	*Semester II*
Organic Chemistry	Medical-Surgical Nursing
Anatomy and Physiology II	Nursing Communication
General Psychology	Systems of Health Care
Sociology II	SENIOR YEAR
English II	*Semester I*
Interpersonal Relationships	Pediatrics
SOPHOMORE YEAR	Nursing Research
Semester I	Strategies for Change
Microbiology	Community Nursing
Pathophysiology	*Semester II*
History	Obstetrics
Humanities	Psychiatric Nursing
Semester II	Nursing Leadership
Nursing History	Nursing Elective
Humanities	

If some nursing schools were to try this on an experimental basis, the response would probably be overwhelming. Hopefully, the demand for such courses would spread throughout nursing's educational process.

Table 2-5 relates the typical Master's program for nurses. Instructors in these programs could effectively introduce a curriculum about private practice into any of the three semesters.

The first semester course entitled Human and Environmental Matrices of Nursing would accommodate lectures on private practice. In the second semester, many locations are available: Curriculum Development, Delivery Systems of Nursing Services, or the elective course are good areas to include instruction on private practice. In the third semester, the Nurse as an Advocate or Nursing Research are two areas where it would fit.

Remember that in any of the areas of concentration, the actual clinical setting should be a private practice. Students may want to develop an

Table 2-5 Typical Curriculum of a Master's Program in Nursing

Nursing Program

First Semester	Area of Concentration
Family Development	Area of Concentration
Science of Man	Elective
Group Behavior	*Third Semester*
Statistics	Nursing Research
Human and Environmental	The Nurse as an Advocate
Matrices of Nursing	Area of Concentration
Second Semester	Area of Concentration
Curriculum Development	Independent Study
Delivery Systems of Nursing	
Service	

independent study concerning the topic. This is an excellent chance for students to exercise their creativity.

Hopefully the Doctoral candidate would have had significant exposure to private practice before his or her entry into a doctoral program for nursing. The study could be included at this level but probably is best at the lower levels so that it is within reach of a greater number of nurses.

Nursing School Philosophy

Along with curriculum changes in education come changes in the purpose, philosophy, or objectives to which nursing schools adhere. Exhibit 2-1 illustrates the typical purpose, philosophy, or objectives of a vast majority of nursing schools in the country.

The philosophy described in Exhibit 2-1 clearly states that nurses are professional practitioners who must implement changes in their profession. Furthermore, this philosophy states that the faculty wishes to prepare general nurse practitioners who will make continuing contributions to the profession. This confirms that the need to incorporate teaching about an alternative modality to traditional delivery of health care is largely the responsibility of the nursing profession and its educational institutions.

WHY AREN'T NURSING SCHOOLS TEACHING PRIVATE PRACTICE?

What, then, is each nursing school waiting for? Are they concerned over the legalities of teaching private practice? If so, the schools should begin by asking

Exhibit 2-1 Example of Purpose, Philosophy, or Objectives of a Great Many
Nursing Schools

The purpose of this nursing school is to provide an educational environment
that qualifies the graduate to function as a professional practitioner of nursing.
This faculty will prepare generalists who will be self-directing and responsible
for continuing contributions to the goal of delivering optimal health care for
all individuals. Delivery of nursing care will require interaction with other
professionals involved in the patient's care.

The faculty believes that each individual has the right to develop his or her
personal identity and autonomy. Thus, the student must be treated educationally as a unique individual.

The faculty believes that every nurse is professional, able to implement the
nursing process, and genuinely concerned about the quality of health care he
or she delivers to the public. The professional nurse must recognize the relationship of the profession to society and take an active part in creating change
to advance the technology of the modality in which nursing is delivered.

---

their state education departments for clear guidelines on a proposed curriculum with a phase of instruction on private practice. Perhaps each nursing
school is waiting to see what the other is going to do; perhaps schools are not
offering these courses because they hold some of the assumptions about private
practice outlined in Table 2-1.

Probably what is really occurring is that the dean or principal of the nursing
school and the faculty are mistakenly believing incorrect assumptions and
failing to investigate them fully. The deans and principals of nursing schools,
as nurses, probably practice much as those above them on the career ladder
did. These people often make meaningful decisions and contributions in the
education process, and they are reluctant to try something innovative.

Considerations To Be Taught

When students are taught the mechanism of private practice, it must be
stressed that they never forget to obtain a physician's order, when needed, and
to always perform nursing care they can correctly and safely perform. They
should obtain assistance as needed. This entire safety mechanism of:

- obtaining physician's orders as needed
- recognizing and not giving care you cannot provide
- obtaining assistance as needed

is taught over and over throughout the levels of nursing education—Funda-mentals, Medical-Surgical, Pediatric, Obstetrical, and Psychiatric Nursing. Not only is it taught in these areas of study but also in specialty areas and in all the clinical settings. The instructor must reinforce this safety mechanism while teaching private practice in the new clinical setting, a nursing practice, or in the classroom.

Nursing schools are currently teaching their graduates to practice the profession of nursing as a registered professional nurse. The actual practice of nursing is defined as performing service in the maintenance of health, prevention of illness, and care of the sick. This requires the nurse to practice principles of nursing based on the biological, social, and physical sciences learned in nursing school. Nurses will supervise and actually provide nursing care and treatment through observation of their clients' condition; they will record these conditions and practice appropriate nursing measures. Carrying out physicians' orders for treatment and medication will also constitute nursing practice.

What are appropriate nursing measures? A later chapter discusses schedules of nursing services, listing many types of nursing measures.

Curriculum Philosophy

Curriculum philosophy of many nursing schools is similar to the one in Exhibit 2-2.

This type of a curriculum philosophy easily accepts the private practice concept because the student upon graduation will be prepared to practice nursing at all three levels. Students in nursing schools that implement curriculums with education about private practices for nurses would bring their nursing skills into private practice as a graduate nurse. The graduate nurse's functions are the same when caring for clients from a private practice as in providing care in traditional settings.

THE NURSING SCHOOL AS THE CHANGE AGENT

The nursing school is a powerful source of change because of its influence on new practitioners. A major breakthrough would occur if some nursing schools offered this type of education in their curriculums.

Epstein explains that Dr. Mayhew contends that higher education is a social institution seeking to achieve goals assigned to it by society. This has been true in nursing almost to the point of fanaticism. When society speaks, nursing jumps. Nurses are responsive to the desires of health care institutions and other health care professionals, primarily physicians. Only recently have nurses

Exhibit 2-2 Example of Curricular Philosophy of Many Nursing Schools

The curriculum of this nursing school is based on a framework of preventive nursing intervention focusing on three levels of care. These levels of care include nursing intervention at the primary preventive, secondary preventive, and tertiary preventive levels.

The primary preventive level is nursing at a level of health care delivery that centers on the maintenance of optimal health of the public at all developmental stages. Our graduates will have learned the skills and knowledge to discriminate a healthy person from an ill person and to recognize a person's behavior as an indication of illness.

The secondary preventive level is nursing care that promotes health while tuning into an illness of an individual at all stages of development. Our students, upon graduation, will have the knowledge and skills to identify illness and the ability to formulate nursing practice plans to promote the health of that person.

The tertiary preventive level is nursing care that promotes health, focusing on the return to optimal health for the individual. Upon graduation, the student will have the knowledge and skills to assess a person's health status and the ability to practice nursing, returning clients to their optimal level of health.

---

begun to consider determining their own direction or exerting influence on the direction of health care delivery. Thus nurses are attempting to change their educational process of generic nursing education.

As educators, we mourn the passivity of nurses and their subservience to physicians and the health care system. Nurses rigidly adhere to tradition. Nurses hope and expect the new liberally college-educated graduates will be our change agents. Nurses are trying to redefine their professional identity and roles. More self-direction, autonomy, independent judgment making, and increased spheres of responsibility should be strived for. Nursing needs greater control of nursing. Data indicates that nursing students entering colleges of nursing tend to have high nurturence and deference levels and very low levels in autonomy and achievement. Thus it may be difficult to achieve a different set of values in nursing without a purposeful effort.[17]

Epstein further states that an object of curriculum change is the modification of the behavior and attitudes of students with resulting changes in institutions and agencies for nursing.

The changes involve attitudes and behavior integrated around the self. These imply giving up something to which the person is committed and values. Changes of this sort tend to be resisted. The proposal of change implies that previous behavior and attitudes were wrong, a conclusion no one wants to acknowledge. Change involving students, faculty, administration, community resources, or hospitals is resisted by the people involved.[18]

Motivating for Reform

An award could be given at nursing school graduations reflecting the activities of graduates in private nursing practice. An award such as "The Most Potential Private Nurse Practitioner" could be provided by nursing schools. The nursing profession could thus begin changing its thinking and encourage its future members to become more aware of private practice. It would motivate and obtain change as well as allow the schools of nursing to be change agents.

Nursing schools, whether or not they have a course in private practice, should make such awards available to their graduates. The criteria for such an award could include several of these:

- self-motivation
- eagerness and ability to develop advanced nursing skills
- ability to practice nursing safely when not directly supervised
- ability to accept role transfer
- a high level of responsibility
- ability to take a risk
- more than adequate communication skills
- problem solving ability
- past or present interest in private nursing practice

In order for changes to occur in nursing or in nursing education, there must first be someone who wants to bring about a change and who sees in this change an improvement. The next requirement is that a general feeling, at least, exist on the part of a number of individuals that they, too, want change and see it as an improvement. Yet another key factor for change to occur is that an administrative and significant person believe sufficiently in the change to be willing to implement it.

There is one other requirement for change to occur. One or more individuals must promote the change, and they must have the skills or the potential to implement it. This text is important for self-study in the event you cannot obtain formal education about private practice.

Syllabus for Private Practice

Table 2-6 depicts a suggested syllabus for a course in private practice for nurses. This course could be included in a vast majority of current curriculums in nursing schools throughout the country. Each school, depending on its level of graduate, may have to alter the suggested curriculum somewhat. This syllabus may be utilized for an undergraduate or graduate level; the depth of the lecture content and clinical exposure may be the primary difference. The primary goal of the syllabus is to expose the student to this modality of practice.

After completing generic nursing education, the novice nurse enters nursing on the first rung of nursing practice. As the novices acquire didactic and clinical skills, they become more proficient, moving from the lowest rungs to higher levels of sophisticated practice. Not all nurses are capable of progressing from this first level of nursing, says Rosasco.[19]

After completion of a course in private practice some nurses could progress into the sector of private practice. It must be strongly restated that private practice is not for all nurses. However, all nurses should have information and courses available to them so that they can determine this for themselves.

Christman feels that nurses should understand that graduation and licensure represent more than an entry to practice. They represent a mandate to continued education. Professional practice means a lifetime of learning. This lifetime of continuing education is not necessarily a 40-hour week.[20]

SUMMARY

Nurses should possess current knowledge of the procedures that enable clients to return to their homes and community while they still require close nursing and possibly some medical supervision. This knowledge will encompass many areas of nursing services. Not only must nurses understand the physiological effects of their clients' conditions but also the emotional impact on the client, family, and community; nurses must be ever aware of the adjustments they have to make to assure quality of life.

As more people choose to live out their lives in familiar surroundings rather than in institutional settings, the nurse practitioner must assist the client, family, and community in accepting this change. Nurses and private nurse practitioners need to be taught to manage these changes. This education should be rooted in the generic nursing school level.

Private nurse practitioners will often make decisions affecting the well-being of clients in their practice. It is imperative that nurses possess many skills

Table 2-6 Suggested Syllabus for a Course in Private Practice for Nurses

School of Nursing
Semester
Date

Theory Objectives	Content	Clinical Objectives
To understand more fully what private practice is and to be cognizant of the terms and history relating to it	I. Private Practice a. definition b. terminology c. history	The student will be able to conceptualize private practice.
To have knowledge of the many positive objectives of nursing practice	II. Private Practice Objectives and the Community a. the nurse as a provider b. lower cost of health care c. reduce overcrowded conditions in hospitals, doctors' offices, and emergency rooms d. increase availability of nursing care to the public e. enhance the profession of nursing as a profession	The students will be able to implement these positive objectives into their practice if they choose to enter one.
To make the student cognizant of several types of nursing care and how these relate to private practice	III. Nursing Care Available in Private Practice a. types of care b. types of care not provided c. a general practice d. a specialized practice	The student will be capable of entering private practice upon becoming licensed and will have a useful number of nursing care procedures available for clients.
To raise the level of consciousness regarding regulations of private practice	IV. Regulations a. assumptions b. prerequisites c. safety d. definition of nursing practice e. the nurse and the law f. malpractice insurance g. records	The students will realize the legal implications when considering opening their practices.
To understand the many facets of referrals	V. Referrals a. sources b. how generated c. to yourself d. to others	The student will have the skill and knowledge to make adequate and professional use of referrals.

To develop an understanding regarding the instruments that make up private practice	VI. Equipment a. purchasing b. layout c. choice	The student will be able to make skillful use of equipment and the finances to purchase it.
To provide an understanding of the costs, business decisions, and laws governing business. Also this prepares the nurses to accept payment from the patient on a fee-for-service basis and raises awareness of various insurance plans and how they relate to nurses as providers.	VII. The Business Process a. finances b. location c. making the public aware of your practice d. insurance plans and fee schedules e. fee-for-service f. business laws as related to professionals g. researching community needs	The student will have a body of knowledge gained from an actual nursing practice (clinical setting) that relates to the subject matter in this content. The students will have the knowledge to decide if private practice is desirable to them.
To allow the students to examine their feelings about their personal capabilities to practice this way. This content also enables the students to *further* understand the needs of their community.	VIII. The Challenge a. nursing dichotomy b. transfer of responsibility c. are you ready for private practice? d. nursing is ready for private practitioners; is the community?	After being involved in a nursing practice as a clinical setting, the student will understand and will have seen the community's needs. This student will also be able to appreciate the true potential of the profession.

enabling proper judgment about clients' care. The nurse practitioner must be cognizant of community resources that can help meet the needs of the client or family.

It behooves the educational facilities to be aware of the skills needed to function in the community and to provide an education that enables the student to learn and grow. By doing this, the nursing profession will learn and grow, meeting the needs of the public. When nursing education and nursing service join forces to prepare knowledgeable nurse practitioners, a greater public service goal will begin to be met.

Formal education is perhaps the most direct pathway toward preparing nursing's practitioners for private practice. However, private practice skills and knowledge can be acquired through self-study or continuing education. The latter educational pathways are as professional and current as the formal pathway. Self-study and continuing education provide skills and knowledge for those nurses already practicing.

NOTES

1. Patricia Rooney McAtee, R.N. and Henry K. Silver, M.D., "What About a National Nurse-Practitioner Program?" *RN* 38, no. 12 (December 1975): 23.

2. M. J. Cutler, "Nursing Leadership and Management: An Historical Perspective," *Nursing Administrative Quarterly* 1 (Fall 1976): 7.

3. William C. Fowkes, Jr. and Virginia K. Hunn, *Clinical Assessment for the Nurse Practitioner* (Saint Louis: The C. V. Mosby Company, 1973), p. 1.

4. Judith L. Sateren and Devra E. Westover, "Baccalaureate Preparation for Action-Practice Nursing," *Nurse Educator* 3, no. 5 (September-October 1978): 12.

5. Carrie B. Lenburg, "Bicentennial Forecast: Nursing Education," *RN* 39, no. 3 (March 1976): 21.

6. Elsie Simms, "Preparation for Independent Practice," *Nursing Outlook* 25, no. 2 (February 1977): 114.

7. Edythe Alexander, *Nursing Administration in the Hospital Health Care System* (Saint Louis: The C. V. Mosby Company, 1972), p. 61.

8. *Ibid.,* p. 118.

9. Dorothy D. Aeschliman, R.N., M.S., "A Strategy for Change," *Nurse Practitioner* 1, no. 3 (January-February 1976): 121.

10. Thelma M. Schorr, R.N., ed., "Meeting in Minneapolis," *American Journal of Nursing* 73, no. 7 (July 1973): 1203.

11. William C. Fowkes, Jr. and Virginia K. Hunn, *Clinical Assessment for the Nurse Practitioner* (Saint Louis: The C. V. Mosby Company, 1973), p. 2.

12. Thelma M. Schorr, R.N., ed., "Meeting in Minneapolis," *American Journal of Nursing* 73, no. 7 (July 1973): 1198.

13. Patricia T. Haase, "Pathways to Practice—Part I," *American Journal of Nursing* 76, no. 5 (May 1976): 809.

14. Susan L. Jones, R.N., Ph.D. and Paul K. Jones, Ph.D., "Nursing Student Definitions of the 'Real' Nurse," *Journal of Nursing Education* 16, no. 4 (April 1977): 20.

15. Barbara Ellis, "Nursing Profession Undergoes Intensive Scrutiny and Adjustment," *Hospitals, J.A.H.A.* 517, no. 7 (April 1, 1977): 142.

16. Elsie Simms, "Preparation for Independent Practice," *Nursing Outlook* 25, no. 2 (February 1977): 118.

17. Rhoda B. Epstein, "Focus on Nursing Education," *Proceedings—Open Curriculum Conference IV* (New York: National League for Nursing, September 22–23, 1975), p. 19.

18. Ibid., p. 18.

19. Louise C. Rosasco, "Of Nursing Practice and Nurse Practitioners," *Nursing Digest* (May-June 1975): 37.

20. Luther Christman, "Accountability and Autonomy Are More Than Rhetoric," *Nurse Educator* 3, no. 4 (July-August 1978): 6.

Chapter 3

Continuing Education, Self-Study, and Consultation as Pathways to Private Practice

PATHWAYS

Pathways refer to how a practicing nurse can acquire knowledge for entry into private practice. Nurses who want further information about private practice have three fairly accessible pathways to finding out what private practice is all about:

1. continuing education
2. self-study
3. consultation with a nurse in private practice

The direction of change lies in the hands of the nursing profession's members. It is in their power to change their professional role, if they wish. Today, articles in trade journals discuss change in this profession. Individual nurses can be more aggressive change agents.

Currently, traditional employment institutions for nurses are easily entered, widely accepted, expected, and taught in nursing school. Nurses, if they truly want to implement change, must develop new avenues to reach the public. This change can be accomplished through private practice, either in a group or as an individual. Private practice helps health care and disease prevention to reach more people.

The nurses who enter private practice can aid the public on a desirable, one-to-one basis. Through private practice, the public obtains direct access to professional nurses.

Traditional Institution Restrictions

At this time nurses' services are in great demand. Institutions are not hiring enough nurses to meet the public's needs. Current institutional employment settings restrict the time nurses are able to spend with clients. Nurses in these settings are not afforded time to teach clients nor to acquire new skills and knowledge of new procedures. Further, they are discouraged from greater collaboration with physicians. Institutions must restrict nurses from providing a great deal of client care because there is a shortage of nurses in large institutions. Nurses are immobilized by institutional bureaucracy, and nurses restrict themselves by insisting on working in traditional institutions.

Meyer says that tradition-bound disciplines, such as the health care field are undergoing examination—both internal and external. These disciplines are struggling to meet the challenges of educating professionals to cope with the demands of a technical and complex society.[1]

Continuing Education

The availability of continuing education, consultation from nurses in private practice, and self-study should enable many nurses to obtain valuable data about private practice. This information would enable them to make a meaningful decision as to whether they want to enter private practice, or whether they are capable of it. The data currently available should give them enough exposure to begin managing their own private practices.

Continuing education programs offer continuing education units or credits. These units become a permanent record of your participation; they are filed in the providing agency. Most programs are designed to meet the educational interests and practice needs of nurses. Courses are open to all nurses unless specific prerequisites are stated in the course description.

Nurses receive certificates for satisfactory completion of programs according to contact hours approved by the official state office. Usually the agency providing the continuing education welcomes the opportunity to discuss training needs with the consumers of its service. Often the agencies are prepared to offer appropriate courses, conferences, in-service workshops, and consultation services to meet these needs.

According to Mote, continuing education must be viewed as a means of ensuring high-quality care. Methods must be developed and employed to measure the impact of continuing education on job performance. Continuing education must not become a circus of conferences, workshops, lectures, and conventions that are funded at the clients' expense. Continuing education must have a direct influence on the quality of client care. This would justify its costs.[2]

Continuing Education and the Nursing School

Usually nursing schools are the agencies that offer continuing education for nurses. Nursing schools generally require a participant in the program to be a citizen or national and a nurse. Traditional institutions where nurses are employed may also offer continuing education about private practice.

Courses provided in these continuing education programs might be set up as two-day workshops, weekend conferences, six Wednesdays between 5:00 and 7:00 in the evening, or one-day experiential conferences.

A nationwide standard of measurement has been proposed for these continuing education programs: the continuing education unit (CEU). The CEU is defined as ten contact hours of participation in an organized continuing education experience under responsible sponsorship, capable direction, and quality instruction. The CEU earned per various courses may, for example, be anywhere from 0.3 CEU to 2.5 CEU, depending upon the amount of credit hours.

A Course in Private Practice

Table 2-6, entitled "Suggested Syllabus for a Course in Private Practice for Nurses," could be implemented easily into any continuing education program. The entire course given would cover private practice; sections of it would offer nurses the option of studying the course at various time intervals or of taking only certain sections. There may be no need to stipulate that all of the sections be completed before credit is issued or before entering private practice, because nurses can obtain needed information from sources other than courses.

The reason for splitting this course into sections would be to meet the needs of the nurses; it should be suited to nurses' working hours, family obligations, and life styles. Nurses who complete all of the sessions of the course could gain a fuller understanding of private practice and receive the full complement of CEU credits. Each section of such a course could offer partial CEU credit.

Continuing Education in Traditional Institutions

Traditional institutions employing nurses have continuing education programs that are developed in the In-Service Education Department. Private practice could be a topic introduced in order to educate and increase employee awareness of private practitioners and the care they provide. A general awareness of private practice would permit a flow of information that would facilitate referrals and consultations between the health care deliverers. Possibly more knowledge about private practice and a direct visit to one would encourage some nurses to enter private practice.

Teaching about private practice clearly is not intended to work against traditional institutions of health care delivery. Private practice is meant to enhance nursing care to the public by working towards the same goal as these institutions: to prevent illness and restore health. Communication should be open between the established institutions and the new ones, nursing practices.

The bureaucracies that employ nurses have been examples of authoritarian control, says Ramphal. Nurses as a group have been subject to the usual bureaucratic controls exerted over salaried professionals and to the charismatic authority system of another profession, medicine. Frequently, hospital administration and medicine join forces to deprive nursing service of any degree of professional autonomy. Even in bureaucratic terms, the director of nursing is within a narrow and perilous channel of decision making caught between medicine and administration.[3]

Nursing is held back from autonomy by other disciplines and by some of its own leaders. While a course on private practice for nurses would fit easily into most in-service education departments, motivating nurse educators to prepare and deliver the course is frequently difficult.

Fromm discusses her first job at a community hospital; she looked forward to a tough orientation program. Instead, she found an ancient In-Service Education Department that spent more time going to and coming from coffee breaks than teaching. Specific orientation to individual areas of specialization had not yet been heard of. Thus nurses who would soon be functioning in maternity, pediatrics, or ambulatory service were oriented only to medical-surgical floors.[4]

Self-Study

A nurse's education must be lifelong in order to maintain true professionalism. Much of this education is obtained through self-study, on-the-job training, or reading trade journals (professional nursing magazines). Entering private practice requires some sort of responsible study.

At the meeting in Minneapolis where the National League for Nursing (NLN) held its 1973 convention, many platform speakers discussed education of all types for nursing. These participants recommended ways nurses could improve their education and patient care.

As a result of the sessions on "Interdisciplinary Education and Practice," it was recommended that a wide variety of instructional experiences in other disciplines be provided nurses at all levels. Interdependent client care activities should be identified, and continuing evaluation should be provided to reduce fragmentation of care. Participants suggested that NLN and the National Student Nurses Association hold joint conferences to encourage pilot projects in interdisciplinary education. Nurse faculty members should also work more closely with physicians in clinical settings to provide role models for students, Schorr explained.[5]

Responsible instruction before entering private practice includes self-study. The motivated nurse can obtain this by reading trade journals and textbooks on the subject. Nursing trade journals include packets for self-study; the syllabus and its content offered in Table 2-6 would be an excellent starting point for periodicals that want to set up a program of instruction about private practice. The content of that syllabus is developed throughout this text.

Connie L. Curran, in her article "What Kind of Continuing Education?" in *Supervisor Nurse*, volume 8, no. 7, July 1977, page 72, prepared a survey of nurses in six Chicago-area hospitals regarding their participation in several types of continuing education. Fifty-six percent reported reading professional literature for one hour a week. The fact that more than half of the nurses read professional literature only one hour a week and that over 40 percent did not attend workshops in the preceding year paints a dismal picture regarding voluntary participation in continuing education activities by employed nurses, according to Curran.

Hopefully this characteristic will not apply to nurses in the future. Curran explains in her article that while specific learning needs of each nurse may vary, a knowledge gap exists that nursing must strive to bridge. The rapid changes occurring in all aspects of the health care delivery system are widely recognized. Nurses must actively participate in continuing education activities to remain current and competent in their practice.

Self-study is logical and accessible to a vast majority of nurses. It is a useful pathway for study of any aspect of the nursing profession, provided the individual nurse utilizes the material properly.

Consultation

The technique of nursing consultation is a pathway to opening a private practice and an excellent mechanism. Although it is actually a form of self-study, it merits separate discussion because it is unique.

Consultation as a method of learning more about something you want to know about is a technique everyone uses daily on a small scale. It can be a conversation, and at this level it is neither costly nor time consuming. Often informal consultation will give you information for your private practice. This method is truly invaluable. Consultation with others, not necessarily nurses, is a great tool for discovering many little, but important, facts before and after opening private practice. Table 3-1 suggests some people with whom you may want to consult.

Table 3-2 provides a guide to people with whom you may want to consult in a formal and official sense. At this level the consultation will take more time, and there may be a fee for the consultant's time.

Table 3-1 Good Sources for Informal Consultation

1. *Nurses*—ask co-workers and friends for advice on opening a private practice and find out if they will assist you, become involved with you, or refer clients to you.
2. *Friends*—ask their advice and find out if they will provide moral support and assistance as needed. Plant a seed of thought for them to visit you and refer others to you.
3. *Physicians*—obtain advice from co-workers and friends on opening a private practice. Ask them to consult with you later and to refer clients to you.
4. *Pharmacists*—find a cooperating pharmacist who will work with you by providing medications for your clients and supplies and equipment for your practice. Pharmacists are an excellent referral source.
5. *Medical Supply Houses*—find one from whom you can purchase supplies for your clients and supplies or equipment for stocking your practice. Ask the personnel for suggestions and referrals.
6. *Landlords*—find out about rent costs, laws governing private practice, and landlords' willingness to allow your practice in their building.
7. *Real Estate Brokers*—find out about local rent costs and laws governing private practice.
8. *Town Hall*—become aware of local ordinances governing where professional nursing practices can be located, what type of shingle (sign) can be legally hung, and any other data they may have to offer.
9. *Significant Others*—be ready to make conversation spontaneously with anyone you come into contact with to obtain advice and referrals.

Facts—Formal and Informal Consultation

Formal or informal consultation is a fantastic tool you can easily use to discover needed facts and advice about your practice. Consultation is a two-way street; you use it to seek information for management of your practice and at the same time it becomes an avenue to inform others of your service.

Your entire presentation at these consultations is extremely valuable, since you will be examined by them. They will be determining your professionalism, credibility, and capability. At these consultations you will sell your practice while you seek information. If you present yourself well, people will visit your practice, because it is you they see, trust, and communicate with.

Consulting with others will cost time and energy. It is not extremely difficult, but it is something nurses do not usually do. Consultation will enable you to make better judgments about your business and your client care. You will need to learn to make decisions that you have never before faced.

Table 3-2 Good Sources for Formal Consultation

1. *Private Nurse Practitioners*—discuss your practice and listen to the advice given. Seek their suggestions, and utilize them as indicated in your practice. Ask them to refer clients requiring care that you specialize in and that they do not.
2. *Lawyers*—discuss your practice as questions arise. Also, obtain data related to the area of nursing and private practice.
3. *Physicians*—discuss and explain your practice so they will refer clients, trust you, and not feel threatened by you. Seek advice about fee schedules and business practices; open up communication.
4. *Continuing Education Providers*—visit institutions that offer continuing education courses in private practice. You may want to take the courses and consult with the instructors.
5. *Nursing Schools*—visit nursing schools that provide courses in private practice. Taking the courses and consulting with the instructors may prove beneficial.
6. *Health Care Delivery Agencies*—visit and consult with the Public Health Department, visiting nurses associations, clinics, hospitals, and other agencies that deliver health care. Explain your role, seek their advice, and let them know your practice is available to assist them in delivery of health care. Explore the possibility for referrals between your practice and their agencies.
7. *Local Nursing Associations*—explain your role, seek their advice and their members' referrals. Let them know you are opening your practice to be an adjunct to current forms of health care delivery.
8. *Local Community Groups*—seek to understand their health care needs, and explain your practice so that they may utilize it. Their advice, suggestions, and questions will aid you greatly.

Physicians and businessmen use consultation techniques frequently. Nurses are not aware of this because they rarely see or use it. Nurses come and go from the hospital like clockwork and are not often willing to take on the responsibility of consultation.

In the past nurses were hesitant to spend the time or money to better themselves and their profession. This has been one of the major problems in nursing; hopefully it will change. The costs of consultation are considered start-up costs. This expense will taper off once your practice becomes a going concern.

Personal Consultation Experiences

My period of data gathering before opening my practice and during the first few months after opening was a time I consulted with as many people or agencies as possible. There was a sense of excitement and a goal to find out as many facts as possible to manage my practice legally and to meet the public's needs.

Many physicians provided their valuable time. Believe it or not, some nurses were extremely critical of the practice and me. Support was anticipated from them, but very little was provided by local peers. Some nurses suspected me of wanting to get rich, practicing medicine, using fraud with third-party payers to double or increase bills, and practicing illegally. One such nurse, a supervisor in a local hospital, visited the practice one day to consult with me, explaining that she wanted to open a practice. We talked for hours; then she accused me of practicing illegally as a nurse, of practicing medicine, and of being a charlatan. After showing her the letter from the Secretary of the State Board of Examiners of Nurses in my state demonstrating legality, my nursing license, and offering her the phone to call the secretary, she became very upset and walked out in distrust, not seeking further validation.

In the beginning months it was difficult to break through this feeling of distrust. Now, years later, the mass media has done much to develop trust in the concept of private practice. Local nurses' attitudes changed in about six months, and today they accept the concept.

In the early months there were many nurses who were interested in learning more about the practice and simply had faith and trust in the concept and me. These nurses quickly became allies. Several helped set up the office and donated some of their personal equipment for use at the office.

There were several times when nurses, either local or from afar, sought consultation. An appointment was made, and we met at the practice. Before they arrived, I explained briefly what would be discussed and that the fee was a modest $25 for however long the consultation lasted. After consultation, some refused to submit the fee, claiming they wanted more data, were unaware of the fee, or thought nurses should consult with nurses for free. This may have been due to their high anxiety level from thinking about this role change. They felt much more data were needed, data they now had to gather from experience. I provided free consultations at times; usually they were brief, informal discussions with nurses.

There were several wonderful experiences with consultation. Nurses who flew in from thousands of miles away for consultation returned home and opened their practices. They sent letters periodically with current data on how their practices were doing. They would phone or mail further questions. I visited three of these practices, located in New Jersey, Maryland, and Colorado. All were doing well.

Nurses should be accountable to the public and keep their practice current. Continuing education, self-study, and consultation are very effective methods that work, provided the nurse is willing to work.

As pointed out by Schorr, argument over which kinds of continuing education are best should cease. A combination of methods should be used, stated Cloace McGill, Director, Continuing Education, University of Texas, San Antonio. Vernice Ferguson, Chief, Nursing Department, National Institutes of Health Clinical Center, added that motivation is the key. Motivation will stem from changes in health care and in society.[6]

The pathway you choose to enter into private practice will not really matter too much. What does matter is that you obtain some information beforehand and that you examine your feelings about it. Be certain you want to nurse in this way and that you will be a competent private practitioner.

When consulting with physicians, Exhibit 4-1, Physician's Questionnaire, is helpful; however, you should develop your own questions as you see the need for them. Also, the Private Nurse Practitioner Questionnaire, Table 6-1, is useful for consulting with private practitioners. Be sure to develop your own questions as needed. It is wise to be prepared with well-thought-out questions before consulting with anyone, especially during formal consultation.

SUMMARY

Independent continuing education can be a viable learning resource to the motivated nurse. Whatever the form, it should be utilized to its fullest extent.

Keeling and Noriega explained that the traditional institutional approach to professional growth raises questions. Can nurses be spared from busy units to attend class? When workshops or classes extend beyond a schedule, can the continued participation of nurses be realistic? Also, is the material relevant to the needs of the unit, institution, and above all, the nurse? Nursing leaders are attempting to provide realistic and workable alternatives to the traditional approach to professional growth.[7]

Nursing should give its members credit and recognition for what they know and what they provide to the public, regardless of whether it was learned in the classroom. E. M. Pattison, in "Residency Training Issues in Community Psychiatry," *American Journal of Psychiatry,* volume 198, no. 9, March 1972, page 1097, observed that the most effective community psychiatry residents were those with the best basic clinical skills. This observation can be carried over into nursing. The most effective private nurse practitioners are those with the best basic clinical skills. These skills lay a foundation of individual competency that carries over into private practice. Motivated and competent nurses will be qualified to provide health care and have the management skills for a private practice after expending time and energy in some form of continuing education.

NOTES

1. Linn Meyer, ed., "Educational Requirements Raise Controversy for Health Personnel," *Hospitals, JAHA* 51, no. 7 (April 1, 1977): 51.

2. John R. Mote, "Continuing Education: Enhancing the Quality of Patient Care," *Hospitals, JAHA* 50, no. 15 (August 1, 1976): 175.

3. Marjorie Ramphal, "Peer Review," *American Journal of Nursing* 74, no. 1 (January 1974): 65.

4. Linda Fromm, "The Problem in Nursing: Nurses!" *Supervisor Nurse* 8, no. 10 (October 1977): 15.

5. Thelma M. Schorr, R.N., ed., "Meeting in Minneapolis," *American Journal of Nursing* 73, no. 7 (July 1973): 1205–1206.

6. Thelma M. Schorr, R.N., ed., "ANA Convention '76," *American Journal of Nursing* 76, no. 7 (July 1976): 1128.

7. Arlene W. Keeling and Lawrence Noriega, "Continuing Education—Independently!" *Supervisor Nurse* 9, no. 4 (April 1978): 45.

Part II

Establishing a Private Practice

Chapter 4

Assessment—The Basis for Determining Community Needs

COMMUNITY ASSESSMENT

The need for better health care in our communities is evident without extensive research. You will realize that it exists if you think about it. The need for better health care is a major theme in news articles. The concept of private practice is applicable to any community; it is not restricted geographically.

Why would a nurse want to enter into private practice when there are so many physicians in it? The first thing to ask is: What are the sources of supply? Are there really so many physicians in private practice that private nurse practitioners are unnecessary?

Probably many physicians' practices are scattered throughout your community. There may seem to be enough physicians in private practice to meet your community's needs. This is how it can appear as you wend your way through your community. Consult with hospital nurses, emergency department (ED) nurses, physicians, and nurses who work for physicians. Consultation may inform you that there is overcrowding and a backlog for health care. Visit waiting rooms of EDs and physicians' private practices to see these crowded conditions for yourself. Examine the distribution and use of health services. A thorough, complete, and lengthy study is not necessary to raise your awareness of the need for additional health care delivery. Nurses could benefit from consciousness-raising about their community's health care needs.

Informal consultation with the public or formal consultation with local community groups should enable you to develop a clearer understanding of the needs of your community and its members. Random phone calls of inquiry to health care providers, health care agencies, or community members may prove useful. While making these telephone inquiries, it would be wise to have a prepared list of standardized questions. This telephone survey should be carried out with complete professionalism and confidentiality.

These fast-moving hours of survey will probably tell you that there is a need for nursing care from private practice. Consulting with other health care providers and going into the community can really inform you of the needs in your community. Field work will also acquaint you with physicians and nurses you may soon be receiving referrals from, referring to, and collaborating with regarding care.

Statistics

Preparations by what was the Comprehensive Health Planning Council and now is the Health Systems Agency (HSA) may be helpful for your assessment. The governmentally established HSAs are located throughout America. They often prepare booklets exploring physician resources and consumer health needs in given communities.

According to Kruzas, local HSAs are established under the provisions of the National Health Planning and Resources Development Act of 1974 (P.L. 93-641). Each HSA is responsible for providing adequate health planning for its health service area and also promoting and developing health care personnel and facilities. State Comprehensive Health Planning Agencies are also established under this law; they operate under state governments.[1]

The Comprehensive Health Planning Council's booklet, entitled (Your County) *Physician Resources,* has many facts and figures from studies on the availability of physicians to population. The following is an example of what is provided:

- physicians per 100,000 persons in your region
- ratio of physicians to population, your region
- your region's physician specialty distribution by town
- population and physician growth in your region
- time spent in direct client care by your region's physicians
- future physician needs related to projected population growth and projected physician growth
- physician shortage by target area
- much more

In my region there were 135.4 physicians per 100,000 people when I opened my private practice. Physician growth was rapid, but so was the population growth. Thus the ratio of physicians to population remained low. The data provided by the local HSA indicated the need for increased provision of health care to the public. As Presser explains, physicians usually locate in medium and large communities. General and family practitioners migrate to communities similar to those they themselves came from, usually to communities of

1–10,000 population. Specialists desire larger communities; generalists desire small communities. In general, communities of less than 1,000 population are not desirable to any physician. Physicians who specialize migrate from small communities to large communities. General practitioners do not leave large communities for smaller communities to the same extent.[2]

Regardless of the geographical distribution of physicians, greater availability of health care remains a need in almost all communities.

Other materials you may find beneficial, also prepared by the HSA, are:

- Annual Implementation Plan for (your HSA region): You can determine your HSA region from this text.
- Health Systems Plan (your HSA region)

The following is cited from the *Annual Implementation Plan for Nassau-Suffolk:* HSA legislation has mandated participation from consumers to plan and deliver health care to the public. They rely on the voluntary contributions from local residents to blend varied experiences into a common guide for improvement of the region's health and health systems. Local residents' viewpoints and motivations are extended into these preparations.

HSAs are interested in protecting the rights of health care consumers. Human rights recognize the client as a person with individualized social, psychological, cultural and family backgrounds, which relate to that person's health status and care needs. Legal rights include, for example, those determined in the Rehabilitation Act of 1973 (P.L. 93-112), The Education For All Handicapped Children Act (P.L. 94-63), and the Developmental Disabilities Act (P.L. 94-103).[3]

You may want to become involved with your HSA in its planning of health care. Its printed material is available to you upon request. These preparations will support the need for private nursing practice and aid in community assessment to determine community and clients' health care needs. Review of this material, field work, and consultation will also inform you of community and client needs.

A medium-size local public library can be a tremendous aid in your community assessment. Several materials that may be available are:

- *Medical and Health Information Directory* by Anthony T. Kruzas, Editor, Gale Research Co., Book Tower, Detroit, Michigan, 48226, (1977)

This guide covers state, national, and international organizations involved with health care. Government agencies, such as HSAs, educational institutions, health care delivery agencies, information centers, and Professional Standards and Review Organizations are included.

- *American Medical Directory, Geographical Register of Physicians* by Ernest B. Howard, M.D., Executive Vice President, American Medical Association, 535 North Dearborn St., Chicago, Illinois, 60610, (1974), 26th Edition

This directory of physicians in America, the Canal Zone, Puerto Rico, and the Virgin Islands contains data from physicians and other sources. Physicians are listed by address.

- *Directory of Medical Specialists* by the American Board of Medical Specialties, Marquis Who's Who, (1977) 18th Edition, Marquis Who's Who, Inc., 200 E. Ohio St., Chicago, Illinois, 60611

Names of physicians and their addresses are listed according to specialty. Territory covered is America, Canada, and foreign.

- Directory of Community Services, prepared by your community, should be available at your library, from your HSA, or from a community organization.

These directories catalog local services and what they provide.

- Your local Medical Society Directory

Most communities have medical societies or associations, which usually prepare directories with local physicians listed by address and specialty.

These references may be used to contact agencies and physicians for consultation or to mail questionnaires. The public and nursing may benefit by encouraging publications that list physicians, specialists, and societies. You may wish to purchase some of them for use in your practice.

Questionnaires

To further establish community needs of health care, you may want to provide physicians, clinics, hospitals, nurses, and other health care providers with questionnaires. See Exhibit 4-1, Physician's Questionnaire. Self-addressed, stamped envelopes should be provided in mailings to assure a quick response. Questionnaires acquaint the health care providers with your practice and enable them to utilize it appropriately. Although Exhibit 4-1 is entitled *Physician's* Questionnaire, its contents may be utilized for clinics, hospitals, nurses, other providers, and health care systems.

Exhibit 4-1 Physician's Questionnaire

Your address

Physician's address

I am opening a private nursing practice to assist you in the care of clients. I will be available to make home visits to clients or have them visit my practice. Either way, I would collaborate with you regarding the care that is needed and keep you informed of the client's progress.

The client will reimburse me directly.

This practice will save you time, relieve overcrowded waiting rooms, and provide a pleasant service to clients.

You may begin to refer clients immediately. Please check the statement below that expresses your future referral, and please take the time to respond to No. 6.

1. Yes, I will refer clients   _____
2. No, I will not refer clients   _____
3. Maybe   _____
4. Please send more data   _____
5. Contact me for consultation   _____
6. What types of care would referred clients usually need?

Sincerely,
Your name
Nurse Practitioner

COMMUNITY NEEDS

Nurses who enter private practice could develop greater autonomy. Working in the community from private practice, you could acquire:

- independent and sophisticated decision making
- interdependence with the health care team
- confidence building
- transfer of responsibility from physicians or other health care institutions
- assertiveness
- in-depth collaboration with physicians

The rewards of private practice may be limitless. These desirable qualities interface to meet the needs of clients in your community. Some of these needs are outlined in Table 4-1.

Far too often nursing gets involved with studies that are too drawn out, too lengthy, and too time consuming. It would be a misuse of money, nurse power, and time to engage the nursing profession in an extensive and exhaustive study to determine community needs. The depth of research demonstrated here should be extensive enough to determine most communities' needs. Obviously clients in communities would have more health care needs met by nurses in private practice.

A sizable amount of current research evaluates the effects of nurse visits to clients prior to cardiac surgery. Presurgical visits can be carried out by nurses in hospitals or by nurses in private practice through home visits. From either setting the nurse would be the socializer and preoperative teacher of the client. Nurses should recognize that they are assessors, initiators, decision makers, and evaluators of client care. Nurses need to be more assertive and begin to implement these roles, according to Mauksch.[4]

Table 4-1 does not delimit community needs to those depicted; it merely lists the needs nurses will probably find to be most in demand.

The needs you observe in your community may define your practice's goals and philosophy. Defining these requirements and making them available to your community demonstrate the professionalism of your practice.

Goals and Philosophy

When I established private practice, it was imperative that I set forth my goals and philosophy. Community members and health care providers were anxious to know them so they could better understand how this private practice could benefit them or their clients. My goals and philosophy were:

- *goals*—To provide a more positive quality of professional nursing care in the community and to meaningfully diversify health care at a lower cost to the consumer. To alleviate the overcrowded conditions in hospital emergency departments and physicians' offices through an innovation in professional nursing. To enhance the availability of health care in our community
- *philosophy*—To maintain health, prevent illness, and care for the sick using the application of nursing principles based on aspects of the biological, physical, and social sciences. To accomplish this by supervising and providing nursing care and treatment through observation, recording, applying nursing measures, and executing physicians' orders. Health procedures will be performed by professional nurses licensed by the authorizing agency of this state.

Your community may benefit if you set goals and philosophies and make them available to the public. You also may benefit as your goals and

Table 4-1 Community Needs

Listening
Teaching about health care
Referral
Helping confused clients to organize health care
Taking blood pressure readings
Giving injections
Removing or changing dressings
Caring for wounds
Reinforcing a health care regime
Evaluating clients' problems
Making a nursing diagnosis
Skillfully establishing a well-thought-out plan of care and implementing and
 evaluating it
Catheter care
Diabetic care
Diet counseling
Checking vital signs
Tracheostomy care
Bowel and bladder training
Emergency care
Rehabilitation
Cast care
Preoperative teaching
Prehospitalization teaching and care
Posthospitalization teaching and care
Assisting with health care
Offering time to clients
Counseling

---

philosophies combined with the community needs will help you to develop the
types of services you should render to your clients.

SUMMARY

Assessment will provide the data that is needed to conceptualize your community's health care system as a whole. Surveying your community may point out deficits, surpluses, ages, use and misuse of health resources, needs of the community as a whole and of its individual members, the demand for private practice, and ways private nursing practice can meet these needs. Reinhardt and Quinn say that:

> the nurse in the community is able to identify needs, to assess priorities for intervention and to plan, implement and evaluate health care services. By making these observations, judgements and implementations, nurses will make meaningful contributions to their communities.[5]

Nurses who enter private practice enter public health. That is, they provide health care to the public. In doing so, the nurse promotes the prevention of disease, the treatment of illness, and public teaching about health care.

Private practice can meet the needs of your community. Nurses can meet the needs of private practice. Experience, education, motivation, collaboration with others, and entry into private practice can meet the needs of nurses. Nurses can safely provide services that clients in the community require and are not yet receiving.

NOTES

1. Anthony T. Kruzas, *Medical and Health Information Directory* (Detroit, Michigan: Gale Research Co., 1977), p. 236.

2. Carole S. Presser, J.D., "Factors Affecting the Geographic Distribution of Physicians," *The Journal of Legal Medicine* 3, no. 1 (January 1975): 15.

3. Nassau-Suffolk Health Systems Agency, Inc., "Forward," *Annual Implementation Plan for Nassau-Suffolk,* January 12, 1978.

4. Ingeborg G. Mauksch, R.N., "Paradox of Risk Takers," *AORN Journal* 25, no. 7 (June 1977): 1308.

5. Adina M. Reinhardt and Mildred D. Quinn, *Family-Centered Community Nursing* (Saint Louis: The C. V. Mosby Company, 1973), p. 179.

Chapter 5

Services Provided and Specialization

DETERMINING WHAT SERVICES TO PROVIDE

To derive the type of nursing care to offer your community, find the nursing care at which you are most proficient that meets the community's needs. Thus, if you are a specialist in psychiatry, you are most capable of delivering quality, safe care in this area. So, psychiatry is your public offering. It would be foolish and unsafe for you to offer nursing care in the surgical area or in the pediatric area. You could offer psychiatric nursing care to pediatric or surgical clients, if they needed psychiatric treatment also. Offer only nursing care in the areas that you can effectively provide. When you yourself cannot provide the care a client requests or needs, you should refer the client to a qualified provider.

Some Clients Require Differentiated Care Contemporaneously

Clients requesting postoperative care for their gastrectomy that was due to an ulcer resulting from diet and/or psychiatric illness will force you to draw on many tools from your nursing background. The mental health nurse practitioner cannot necessarily handle the client's needs alone, in this case. A mental health nurse practitioner is not going to become directly involved with a surgical nurse's role. The surgical nurse specialist or general practitioner will provide the diet teaching, dressings, and possibly some psychiatric care. The family will also need care or support.

According to Pesznecker, as a nurse practitioner you will be actively involved in providing care in the community. You will be in a position to counsel family members and clients who are going through changes in their lives. Counseling of family members can be organized in conjunction with your usual activities. These activities may include health counseling and health education with clients or family members in their homes or at your practice.[1]

Nurses should make referrals to other nurses. The client with the gastrectomy demonstrates a time when two nurse specialists could care for the same client; so could one or more general nurse practitioners if one was proficient in psychiatry and one in surgery.

Ambulatory and Out-Patient Care

Ambulatory or *out-patient* care will be requested from your practice; these two terms do not adequately describe all of the types of care you could offer. Many clients who are nonambulatory may request your care at home after their hospital discharge.

Vital Signs

The cardinal symptoms, or the vital signs, should be taken on all clients with every visit and recorded in nursing notes for that client. This routine is a must.

The vital signs consist of the temperature, pulse, and respiratory rate. It would be a good idea to include blood pressure along with these. These should be compared to the last set in your notes. They tell an important story about the client. From these records, many decisions can be made regarding whether to notify the physician of changes in the client and whether the client is progressing.

Office Visits and Home Visits

Clients and their families can come to your practice by appointment, or visit ad lib during hours. The care required by the client determines the location, either in the office or at home.

Whether an office or home visit (HV) is made, an appointment is best to ensure adequate time for yourself and the client to prepare. The family or the client may telephone you to describe needs, request your aid, and set up an appointment. This gives you time to gather needed equipment, collaborate with the physician, and do research if needed to enhance the quality of care that you provide. Birenbaum contends that the home can be a worthwhile location for care. Families and clients need not be selected for home care according to any special criteria. Developing useful home care depends on the willingness of the health care system. Current health care systems need to reach the public and demonstrate that they can provide services to keep consumers out of hospitals and extended care facilities. Home care is vital in keeping the elderly clients at home and out of old-age homes or nursing homes. Home care can keep disabled children and adults at home, providing appropriate experiences necessary for their growth, development, healing, and overall well-being.[2]

Length of Visit

Nurses and clients complain that physicians rarely afford clients time to ask questions, discuss a problem, or gain information from the physician. Nurses also complain that the nurses themselves do not have enough time with their clients to teach, listen, explain, or provide care. Your private practice can relieve these problems.

Offering clients the amount of time that is necessary or desired is the key. Set a base line of one hour, and adjust it accordingly. Usually after 20 minutes, clients become concerned and ask why you are keeping them. In my experience, time spent with a client after 20 minutes (on an average) made them believe something serious was wrong and was being hidden from them. Never leave the client after 20 minutes if your care is not finished or the client needs your support. Stay until you finish, and the client is able to carry on without you. It is illegal to abandon your clients.

Prepare to stay with your client one hour, but cut the visit short when the client's tension rises. The first visit will probably last a little over one hour while the client and family get to know you. They need this time in the beginning of your relationship.

Schedule of Nursing Services

A typical procedure manual from a ward in an institution would parallel the services offered in private practice. My state nursing association requested an inclusive list of the services to be provided in my private practice. I requested from them a list of services that nurses in that state were allowed to perform. They wrote back explaining that no such list existed, never did, and probably never would. They explained that to prepare such a list would be impossible due to the varied situations nurses encounter. Nurses provide endless types of care or services due to the fact that each client's needs are individualized and unique. Goodspeed, a nurse practitioner, explained that she was plagued by two questions she thought would be constantly asked. The following illustrates those questions and her responses. How do you see yourself in this challenging role? What do you do? The answers were carefully prepared. She stated that she practiced nursing and provided quality nursing care.[3]

Were a schedule of services available from legislation, it would be a guideline for services provided. Hopefully such a list will not be created, as it would restrict diffuse and needed nursing care. Establishing a schedule of nursing services to offer from your practice as observed from your community assessment is a logical and systematic method of defining your task.

Hilary Smith was a nurse in Vietnam, and she cannot understand the problems with role identity in America. She says she never performed a cutdown, started infusions, delivered a baby, lanced an abcess, sutured or debrided a wound. Similarly Smith never performed a spinal tap, paracenthesis, applied a cast, or set up traction. The Montagnards did all these things routinely.[4]

Sometimes nurses grasp at a few comfortable services that make them feel at ease. Nurses should begin to recognize their potential, as they can provide unlimited services. Smith wonders whether the limitations on the Western nurse's role placed by medicine and a sophisticated public aren't responsible for nurses' stubborn clinging to the few prerogatives perceived as left for them.[5]

This text neither attempts to teach development of nursing care plans nor how to provide various nursing services. These should be taught in nursing schools.

Table 5-1 is a schedule of nursing services that can be provided. Table 5-1 does not encompass all of the services nurses may provide; it offers examples of the many services they may offer. You may alter this schedule to meet your needs as well as those of your community and your client.

The Schedule of Nursing Services is a guideline for you, your clients, physicians, and others. An all-inclusive list is not necessary, unless you want to *specifically limit* your practice to special services.

In providing services, it is of utmost importance to use the safety mechanisms described in Chapter 2.

The clients need the care they contacted you for. If you cannot provide it because you are unfamiliar with the care requested or because it is not part of your services, assist the clients by referring them to someone who can.

Nurse specialists could establish their own modified, individualized, and unique schedule of nursing services. Knafl noted that: Student nurse practitioners observed that the individual nurse practitioners held the responsibility to construct their own role. They observed that the nurse practitioners varied in the type, level, and depth of nursing care they practiced. This depended more on each nurse practitioner than on anything else. The nurse practitioners set limits on their professional role to what they were capable of providing and were comfortable with. The individual nurse practitioners had to define their own role boundaries.[6]

Some examples of the areas private nurse practitioners may wish to specialize in are:
- medical nursing
- surgical nursing
- adult nursing
- rehabilitation nursing
- cardiac nursing
- family nursing
- obstetrical nursing
    (*list continues on page 65*)

Table 5-1 Schedule of Nursing Services

*Nursing services are usually available on a same day or by appointment basis.
*Spanish- and English-speaking nurses are available.
*Consult with your physician, and refer as needed.

Services

- alcohol counseling
- drawing blood for laboratory study
- bowel and bladder training
- catheter care:
  a. changing, inserting, and removing
  b. hygienic care
  c. irrigations
  d. explanation and teaching
- child development assessment
- colostomy care:
  a. irrigations
  b. dressing or bag changes
  c. client and family teaching for home care
- diabetic care:
  a. diet therapy
  b. insulin therapy
  c. personal hygiene
  d. exchange diet provided and taught
  e. urine testing
  f. drawing of blood for laboratory analysis
- nutrition counseling (diets explained)
- drug abuse counseling
- limited emergency treatment (Contact nearest emergency department.)
- group therapy
- histories:
  a. nursing observations
  b. nursing diagnosis
  c. physical and neurological status
  d. other
- inhalation therapy:
  a. teaching
  b. breathing exercises
  c. oxygen therapy
  d. respirator therapy
- injections:
  a. taught for self-administration where applicable

  b. given by professional nurses
- drug therapy (prescribed medication):
  a. counseling
  b. teaching self-administration
  c. given by professional nurses
- irrigations:
  a. eyes
  b. ears
- pre- and post-hospital care and counseling
- prenatal counseling and teaching
- postpartum counseling and teaching
- psychosocial counseling:
  a. crisis intervention
  b. one-to-one relationship
  c. interviewing, counseling
  d. referral
- range of motion
- rehabilitation:
  a. assist
  b. support
  c. teach independence
  d. prosthetic care
- suture removal
- tracheotomy and tracheostomy care:
  a. laryngectomy patients
- vision exams:
  a. Snellen's chart
  b. modified Snellen's chart
- vital signs:
  a. temperature, pulse, respirations
  b. blood pressure
  c. management of these
- walker and crutch training
- wound care:
  a. cleansing
  b. applying dressings
  c. teaching personal home care
- stress management
- hypertension control
- obesity control
- counseling students
- interviewing

- referral to:
  a. physicians
  b. agencies
  c. nurses
  d. other health care providers
Care and teaching aspects are oriented to encourage self home care.

(*continued from page 62*)
- gynecological nursing
- pediatric nursing
- midwifery nursing
- geriatric nursing
- psychiatric nursing
- mental health nursing
- psychiatric/mental health nursing
- community mental health nursing
- developmental disabilities nursing
- mental retardation nursing
- mentally handicapped nursing

Schedule of Physicians' Services

Many physicians do not have a schedule of services as elaborate as Table 5-1. Their schedules are often much briefer, such as those posted in waiting rooms with fees attached. Perhaps this is better and more professional. Consult with physicians and ask to see their schedules to familiarize yourself with their services.

Investigating health insurance fee schedules will enable you to understand how the schedule of services is set up for physicians and not for nurses. A health insurance fee schedule is the booklet that explains to consumers what services are insured and who may provide them as well as what services are not covered and by whom.

What Services Not To Provide

It may seem that there is a great deal of care a nurse should be familiar with. The basics to providing most of the care in Table 5-1 should be learned before a nursing student graduates. When practicing privately, it is wise not to become involved with care you are unable to provide or that your practice is not equipped to handle. Some of the services to avoid for the public's safety will now be discussed.

Emergency Care

Regarding Table 5-1, emergency treatment includes only that treatment within your scope to handle. Your private practice is not an emergency department (ED) such as the one in your local hospital.

An emergency department is a place where staff provides emergency care in a setting that contains several nurses and physicians and highly sophisticated equipment. Your practice should not attempt to provide this; it will not have a physician on hand as an ED does. Your practice is not doctorless. However, you, a nurse, manage your practice; you utilize your clients' physicians as needed to enable you to legally and professionally provide client care. You work with clients' physicians when appropriate.

Emergency care is provided to persons coming from the community without an appointment, in need of immediate care. Generally you will not be able to provide this care. But if someone walked in with an injury that needed immediate attention, you would render first aid as emergency care and assist the victim to the local ED. This type of confrontation for emergency care could occur any place.

Transporting Clients to Emergency Departments: You will be able to assist the victim to the local emergency department by several convenient techniques.

First, your community will probably have an ambulance service, either paid or volunteer; it may be incorporated with the fire department. Write the telephone number for it in your office, ready for use, and also record the fire department's telephone number. If a person walked into your office bleeding from a severe wound, you could stop the bleeding, reduce his anxiety, call the ambulance, and assist this person in getting to the emergency department for medical attention.

Second, you could take the victim to the ED yourself or have someone else take him. Each and every emergency case can be dealt with differently. Simply remember to use sound nursing judgement.

Third, keep the police department phone number on hand for emergency aid. They should be willing to assist you in transportation.

Poison Control

Nurses should know something about poison control. Keep the local poison control phone number accessible for immediate use; you never know when you may need it. Part of your equipment could be a poison treatment package, for emergency use. You will not be involved necessarily with pumping stomachs out or giving medications, but you may have to give an emergency antidote as instructed by the poison control center and transport the victim to the ED.

Emergency Care Via Telephone

Community members may call for advice for an emergency: poisoning or injury. Do not necessarily get in your car and go there to provide the care. A better way to deal with this would be to learn over the phone the victim and caller's names, phone number, address, and type of injury; calm the caller; and suggest something to be done immediately. Explain to the caller that you will notify the ambulance, police, or fire department right away.

You could telephone the caller back to provide further instruction as needed and even perhaps alert the ED that an injured person is coming in with whatever type of injury there is, so that it can prepare for the treatment.

Nursing 77, May, has an excellent article on pages 16–20 by Kenneth Emkey, M.D. entitled, "Tempering the Turmoil of an Office Emergency." It is an excellent article, and even though it relates primarily to a physician's office, it makes valuable reading for nurses who enter private practice.

Visits to Nursing Homes

You may consult with local nursing homes and set up a system of fee-for-service payment for you to be on call to visit any hour of the day or night to, for example, change catheters. Also, the nursing home may wish to utilize you as a consultant.

My results with this were not as successful as desired. Nursing homes operate differently, however, and if you canvass enough you may locate one with which you could contract your services.

Hypertensive Screening

Local drug stores may contract with you to provide customers with blood pressure readings on their location. You may post signs one to two weeks in advance notifying the public of the service, listing the inclusive dates, the days of the week, the hours, and the cost.

The cost may be one dollar per reading with explanation and teaching. Customers may come in for free repeat readings; when they have hypertension, refer them to their physician. This can generate meaningful revenue and offer a service to the drug store's clientele, the community members. While doing this, you may inform the community members of your practice.

Referring the Public to Nurses and Physicians

The best way to refer potential clients to a physician, when they do not have one, is to have them choose one from the yellow pages of the telephone directory. Have them call the information operator and ask for one, or you may provide three or more names. Your referrals may derive from the physician sources cited in Chapter 4. If you do not refer to physicians in this manner, you may be looked upon as being oversolicitous to a particular physician, when several exist that are proficient in similar practice. This could leave you open to criticism.

When physicians refer to your office directly, it is acceptable since there probably is not a wide selection of private nurse practitioners. The same is true when you refer to other nurses.

Hot Line

Keep the local hot line phone number handy. Someone may call you seeking information that only the hot line can provide.

Insurance Company Physicals

Many companies that sell life and health insurance contract with local physicians to provide the physical exam required before granting the insurance. The fee paid to the physician is usually about $35 and up. Often exams are able to be performed by a competent nurse. Insurance companies do not ask nurses to provide the exams because nurses have been unavailable, and at times it is important that a physician perform the exam.

To a great deal of proposed insureds, nurses can legally perform the insurance company physicals with the insurance companies' blessings. Insurance companies often prefer nurses because they can get the same physical done for less than what the physician charges. The nurse could make a home visit to the prospective policyholder's home, at this person's convenience. Nurses may be more willing to do these physicals than physicians are.

At any rate, it is up to the nurse practitioner to contact insurance companies to set up a contractual agreement. Visit a local insurance broker and from this broker obtain several addresses for life insurance companies' main headquarters. You will probably obtain better results in seeking to provide life insurance physical exams than health insurance physical exams.

Prepare a letter to the company's headquarters, explaining your practice and your qualifications; include a resume. In this letter clearly explain what you want to do for that company. Recommend a fee per physical; make it lower than what physicians request, for example, $20 as opposed to $35. Find out the fee paid to the physician from the insurance broker and offer the service to the insurance company for less.

You could accept the fee they offer if it is less than what you requested, unless it is demeaning. Accepting a lesser fee is a starting point; you may need to get a trusting, working relationship with the company. The insurance company will usually be glad to contract with you because many physicians are too busy to do these physicals.

Once the insurance company approves you to perform their life insurance physicals for them, they may notify their local agents to refer new customers to you for physical exams.

Not all persons buying life insurance will be able to have their physicals performed by you. Some must be referred to participating physicians. The person that can be examined by nurses may fit into one of the following categories:

- amounts of life insurance up to and including $35,000 and ages through 50. Higher amounts or ages require a physician's exam.
- ages 16–54 purchasing $50,000 in life insurance or less

The company may mail you the necessary forms; these forms will probably contain some information for the physician to complete; delete this area of the form and prepare your part.

Along with the forms from the company will come envelopes, and, most likely, urine containers to enable you to mail the proposed insured's urine samples to their laboratory. Each company may vary slightly; however, this is the basic procedure.

When the company reviews their findings on the urine studies and the information from your exam, they will either approve or disapprove the customer for life insurance. If they approve the customer, your involvement is ended. If they disapprove the customer, the company may ask you to repeat the physical, focusing on a particular area, such as ulcers, blood pressure, and medical history. After receiving this new data, they make another review of the customer.

Sometimes after the first or second review of your data, the company will require a physician to examine the customer in greater depth. This does not mean you did something improper, just that the company wants to know more about their prospective insured before they agree to insure that client.

During this physical exam, nurses could ask the client some of the questions in Table 5-2. When the exam is over, write out the needed explanations, sign the form and mail it, with the urine, to the company after making a copy for your records. Bill the company monthly.

Caring for Clients Who Require Extra Time

Many times, physicians refer clients who need a great deal of time in a one-to-one relationship. This does not mean that physicians do not care to

Table 5-2 Sample Life Insurance Physical Exam Questions

1. Has proposed insured taken or been advised to take medication to control blood pressure?
2. Has proposed insured changed or been advised to change residence or occupation for the benefit of health?
3. Has proposed insured ever had: blood chemistries, x-ray, EKG, EEG ?
4. Has proposed insured been on any special diet for any cause?
5. Has proposed insured ever taken oral antidiabetic agent or insulin?
6. Has proposed insured's urine ever had albumin, casts, pus, sugar, or blood found in it?
7. Has proposed insured ever been treated for alcohol use or a drug habit?
8. Has proposed insured ever had an ailment or disease of:
   a. stomach, intestines, kidneys, bladder, gallbladder, liver
   b. lungs, heart, circulatory system
   c. nervous system or brain
9. Has proposed insured ever been treated for or worked up for:
   a. mental illness or nervous breakdown
   b. enlarged glands, abnormal blood findings, or tumors
   c. epilepsy or convulsions
   d. rheumatic fever, cardiac problem, heart murmur, hypertension, angina pectoris, coronary artery malady, chest pain
   e. unusual or abnormal chest x-ray
   f. any ulcer of the gastrointestinal tract
10. Has proposed insured been under any hospital, asylum, or sanitarium care or treatment, ever?
11. Has there been any suicide, insanity, diabetes, allergies, anemias, leukemias, or epilepsy in the proposed insured's family?
12. Family record: Give age and health of each of the following if living and give age, year of death, and cause of death of the following if deceased:
    a. spouse
    b. father
    c. mother
    d. brothers
    e. sisters
13. Attach sheets of paper as necessary to give detailed and full particulars about illnesses, hospitalizations, diagnoses, and treatments during the last seven years. Also explain yes answers to questions 1 through 11, showing the question number beside the explanation for reference.
14. Blood pressure:
    a. When systolic is over 142 or diastolic is over 90, take additional readings 12 minutes apart.

    b. Blood pressure:
- first reading
- second reading
- third reading

15. Pulse rate:
    a. at rest
    b. after hopping up and down 10 times
    c. two minutes after exercise
16. Any irregular heart beats noted?
17. Mail urine specimen to our laboratory.

---

spend time with clients; sometimes they cannot. When a client is demanding and the physician has an overcrowded waiting room, it is often better for the physician to refer the client to a nurse, who can offer more time for listening and teaching. This benefits the client and the physician, and it allows nurses to receive referrals from physicians in a way that is not threatening. The physician will often gladly refer a demanding client to you in order to give more attention to remaining clients. Clients who insist upon seeing the physician after such a referral should be allowed to do so.

"Patient Dumping: The Big-Clinic Syndrome" is an interesting article in *Medical Economics,* September 5, 1977, pages 269–279, by Mike Oppenheim, M.D. This article, which deals primarily with physicians and their practices, explains that physicians have internal difficulties, and at times need assistance from others. It says that physicians refer difficult clients to one another. If physicians began to utilize the nursing profession more, they might have the time needed to cope with the medically difficult clients. Nurses who would accept physician referrals for these reasons could care for a great number of clients that physicians lack the time for. This could alleviate the physician shortage as nurse and physician roles frequently overlap.

The Overlapping Roles of Nurses and Physicians

Table 5-1, Schedule of Nursing Services, clearly includes many services that are also performed by physicians. Some of these services are even performed by aides or orderlies in hospitals, for example, vital signs, colostomy care, referrals to nurses and physicians, some catheter care, some wound care, and diabetic urine testing. So the thought that roles overlap is not new. Roy and Obloy relate that expanding knowledge and skills for the nurse practitioner include techniques for taking histories and providing physical exams. The development of these skills can be placed in perspective with clients' needs and the nursing model. Not all nurse practitioners have retained a nursing model; many have adopted a quasi-medical model.[7]

CASE PRESENTATIONS

Patients are gained and lost constantly; they become healthier, change providers, move or die. The concept of private practice is to assist existing health care systems, not work against them. The depth of care that the following cases describe will prove informative. About 90% of the author's clients requested care on an HV basis. The following cases demonstrate some of that care.

Joan Hall: Gallbladder Patient

Joan Hall is 46 years old, 141 pounds, five feet five inches tall. Her husband expired three years ago in an automobile accident. She lives at her home with three sons and one daughter.

Her physician contacted the nursing practice as a result of the physician's questionnaire. Her physician requested a nurse to irrigate her T-Tube. The client had just undergone a cholecystectomy and was recovering at home. The physician did a cholangiogram in his office to determine patency of the bile ducts. This office cholangiogram showed a stone in a duct, occluding bile flow into the duodenum.

I pointed out to the physician that this was not a usual procedure for a nurse to practice, but that if the physician were to teach it, I would provide the therapy if I felt competent after the lesson. The physician reviewed the entire case and taught me what to do in his office. Providing the care now was acceptable due to role transfer and a feeling of competence. The physician's written orders were:

1. Irrigate the T-Tube around the clock for seven days.
2. Add 30,000 units of heparin to 250 cubic centimeters (cc.'s) of sterile normal saline, I.V. solution.
3. Run each 250 cc. bottle with the heparin for 6 hours.
4. Teach the client to change the bottles by herself.
5. Visit the client daily.
6. Check the wound. The client changes her own dressing and is on antibiotics due to an infected incision site.
7. Schedule for a repeat cholangiogram on the eighth day.

The reason for this method of treatment (to hopefully dissolve the stone) was to save the client from the insult of a second operation within one month. The physician provided a prescription to enable purchasing the material. An appointment was made with Joan Hall for the home visits.

This client will not hemorrhage as heparin is not absorbed from the gastrointestinal tract. The I.V. tubing is to be attached directly to the T-Tube, the T-Tube is unclamped, and the I.V. runs according to the calculated drop rate for 6 hours per bottle.

The first visit to the client was dramatic. It took about 2 hours to teach her, write down guidelines, and set up for the first 24 hours. The next six visits each lasted 45 minutes, providing vital signs, communication, reassurance, and answering questions she had. She was brave and managed well.

During the first visit, the client's mother walked in while the I.V. began to flow into the T-Tube; she fainted at this sight. The client and I thought she suffered a myocardial infarction. She was examined at once for cardiac output, and it was strong; she had fainted. Her physician was called and wanted to see her that day in his practice. By this time, she was awake and responding.

Joan Hall had a slightly infected incision site but was taking the oral antibiotic prescribed by her physician. The infection cleared up. The irrigation went well except for one day, while she was ironing, the I.V. bottle fell from a nail on the door and broke. Joan clamped the T-Tube, disconnected the I.V. tubing, cleaned up, and started the next I.V. bottle. She told me about it the next morning. I visited Joan Hall each morning, and a nurse was available to her by phone around the clock.

The irrigation was successful, and the fee was only $80 for all seven visits. The equipment cost $60, and her insurance paid for it. This method of treatment kept Joan Hall from repeated surgery. It kept her home with loved ones, in a familiar environment, even though the same therapy could have been provided in the hospital. The costs for this at-home care were less than they would have been in the hospital. Records were kept, and the physician was supplied with a copy.

Alan Davis: Cancer Victim

Alan Davis was a 75-year-old, thin, emaciated man, six feet tall, 110 pounds. He had an ileostomy, leukemia, and Hodgkin's disease. He lived with his wife who cared for him a great deal. She was elderly and unable to go on providing the needed care. The physician referred the client to the private practice. The written orders were:

1. Give Vitamin B_{12}, 1000 micrograms (mcg.), intramuscularly (I.M.) every week.
2. Give ileostomy and stoma care daily.
3. Teach the client about his diet.

This care was provided for a month at the cost of $7 a day, as the client lived within two miles of the nursing practice and, after the first few times, required 30-minute visits.

After two weeks of this care, the client became worse. His physician was notified and out-patient radiation therapy was started. This wore the client out and made him nauseous. He vomited often and became weaker.

The physician ordered him into the hospital for a blood transfusion. Mrs. Davis strongly requested that I administer the blood transfusion at home. The physician consented and wrote the following orders:

1. Give two units of packed cells at home.
2. If there is a reaction, call me for an order to give Benadryl.
3. Have Benadryl 50 milligrams per ampule on hand for push I.V. (10 ampules in all).
4. Have 10 syringes on hand, 10 cc.'s each.
5. Draw blood the day before for complete blood count (CBC) and type and cross match at the local hospital.
6. If the CBC warrants transfusion, administer the two units of packed cells with the type matching the donor blood.
7. Start the procedure by running 100 cc.'s of sterile normal saline into the client first; then piggyback the blood in.

Two physicians signed these orders; they notified the hospital to release the equipment and blood and to perform the tests in #5 of the order. Another nurse witnessed the physicians writing and signing the orders; the client and his wife signed a permit for administration of the blood.

The CBC was low; therefore, the transfusion was to begin the next day. The hospital provided the material and a home visit was made. Before the I.V. was started with the saline, a base line of vital signs was obtained. The I.V. was begun and the blood piggybacked in. The client read a book through the procedure and was constantly monitored. No complications occurred. The procedure was successfully completed at Alan Davis's home without incident.

The fee was $75. The cost of equipment was billed to his insurance company; they paid. The client was kept home and happy. After the procedure, the blood bags and tubing were returned to the hospital laboratory to be tested for infection and to type and cross match their blood again, a safety precaution.

The client was fine for a few months; then he became extremely ill and had to be hospitalized, where he eventually expired. Through the interactions with Mr. and Mrs. Davis, emotional support was provided. Death and dying was a topic they brought up often. A great deal of listening, counseling, and support was provided. Hopefully, they both were comforted. Records were kept, and the physician was provided with a copy.

Robert Alma: Stroke Patient

Robert Alma is an elderly man who suffered a stroke in a distant town. He was institutionalized there in a nursing home. His son lives 20 miles from this nursing practice, and over 1,000 miles from his father. The son flew to his father's side and had his father transported to his home. The son had been caring for his father at home for over one year and eventually called this practice for nursing care. The son called hoping to have a nurse make home visits (HVs) as it was too traumatic to the father (client), son, physician, and clients in the physician's waiting room when this client was wheeled in on a stretcher every two weeks for a suprapubic tube change. The son contacted this practice from the telephone book.

Robert is 85 years old, has a right-sided stroke, cannot talk, can hear well, and responds to conversation. He tries to assist in his care but is not successful. He is six feet tall and weighs 160 pounds. The son feeds, bathes, and provides all other care for his father but wants a nurse to make HVs to check vital signs, make periodic observations, and change the suprapubic tube biweekly.

In conversation with the son on the phone, it was determined that the request could be met. The physician's address, name, and phone number were recorded, and a letter went out to him seeking his approval and orders. A letter was returned shortly from the physician approving of the treatment plan. The orders read:

1. Irrigate suprapubic tube and bladder as necessary with sterile normal saline.
2. Change suprapubic tube as necessary with size 20-5, 22-5, or 24-5 Foley Catheter.
3. Notify me in six months of progress and for possible changes in orders.
4. Notify me at once if needed.

A personal visit was made to the physician to confer on the correct procedure for changing a suprapubic tube. Once explained, there was enough competency to attend to the care.

The needed equipment was brought on the first HV. The son provided reimbursement for this as well as the $25 fee that had been predetermined. The visit fee was determined by the distance traveled, the type of care, and the fact that the HV took over one hour per visit.

Vital signs were always taken, and the client was examined. Observations and vital signs were recorded in nurse's notes. The son talked a great deal about how he gave care to his father. I was able to teach him better techniques where needed and to reassure him that he was doing a good job. Emotional support was provided to father and son as needed.

After a few HVs, the son mentioned that his father was a retired union member. The union was a large national organization that offered its members health benefits, retired or not. While in the home with the client, the son called the union's national headquarters. A discussion followed for about one hour.

Discussion ensued with the person in charge of members' health benefits. A decision was made to reimburse directly, $25 per home visit because this was much less than the physician's charge of $40 and the ambulance transportation cost of $50. This saved the client the trauma of traveling and saved the union a large expenditure every two weeks. The union's pharmacy at its main office would mail needed equipment to the client's home.

The union headquarters sent a packet of payment vouchers to be submitted after each visit. Along with the vouchers was a list of needed equipment. The union mailed by parcel post the catheters, catheter kits, irrigant, chucks, drainage bags, and other equipment at no expense to the client or his son.

The physician was pleased with this plan because he cared about the client and wanted to save him the trauma of being taken from his home every two weeks. Also, the physician was already overworked. The physician's waiting room clients would no longer become frightened by ambulance personnel wheeling in a client.

This therapy regimen lasted only about four months. Vital signs were stable, the physician was continually informed of progress, and everything was going well for the client. Notes were recorded and kept in the files. The union reimbursed immediately with no problem.

The client's son ended this treatment to the client. The son began to become very suspicious of care provided to his father and perceived the nurse's intervention as harmful to his father. Nothing was said or done to make the son feel this way. It was the son's personality. The son asked that this regimen end and sought further help. It was discovered later that this had been a pattern of behavior. The son had gone from physician to physician, eventually unable to trust anyone who provided health care to his father. Several nursing techniques were attempted to help the son, but nothing seemed to work. He simply terminated all interaction.

Betty Jones: Allergy Patient

Betty Jones had been recently married, six months ago. She was three months pregnant and very happy. She telephoned the practice after seeing it listed in the yellow pages of her telephone directory, in the nursing column. Her request was to visit the practice monthly for allergy injections.

An appointment was made; the fee would be $10 per visit. Her physician's name, address, and phone number were established, and a letter was sent to the physician that afternoon. The letter requested the diagnosis and written orders. This letter contained a self-addressed, stamped envelope to expedite receiving orders and diagnosis.

Betty is 24 years old, five feet, nine inches tall, and weighs 128 pounds. She wants to visit the practice because she now travels 30 miles one way to see her physician every month for these injections. This practice is about two miles, one way, for her. Also, the fee per visit is $10 less than the physician's fee, and she does not have to wait in a crowded waiting room.

Her physician mailed approval for this therapy, realizing the trauma of a 60-mile ride for Betty. The orders read:

1. Give Chlor-Trimeton tablets, 4 mg., by mouth 20 minutes before injection.
2. Give one injection monthly. Give ragweed 0.4 mg., trees 0.4 mg., dust and molds 0.1 mg.
3. Give this treatment for six months.
4. When amounts allow, combine the medication in one syringe, properly.
5. Betty Jones' diagnosis is allergy to allergens in item No. 2.
6. She is pregnant, and this therapy is to be maintained.
7. Notify me if any untoward reactions occur.
8. Keep client one-half hour after injection for observation.
9. Notify me in six months for an update on her case and new orders.

The physician confirmed all orders by telephone. Therapy for Betty progressed well. There is a big responsibility when anaphylactic shock may occur at any time. Oxygen was available as well as a tourniquet; Adrenalin 1:1,000 for subcutaneous administration; Adrenalin 1:10,000 for I.V. use as needed; and Benadryl 10 mg. per cc. Regarding the risk of allergic reaction, the physician wrote the following orders:

1. Give adrenalin 1:1,000 subcutaneously for allergic reaction in this manner.
   a. Tie a tourniquet on the arm proximal to injection site and give 0.2 cc. to 0.3 cc. of adrenalin 1:1,000 subcutaneously at the site of injection of allergen and also 0.2 cc. to 0.3 cc. in the opposite arm.
   b. Have the client lie down, and observe constantly.
   c. Repeat the adrenalin every 20 minutes for three to four doses, if needed.
   d. Give Benadryl 10 mg. per cc. I.V. slowly.
   e. Administer oxygen as needed.

There was never a reaction; the physician kept the injected allergen at a safe level to reduce the risk of reaction. If reaction occurred, it would have been treated at once. Vital signs were recorded before, during, and after treatment.

Betty asked for advice and counseling on her soon-to-be-born child. A referral was made to a nurse who belongs to the American Society for Psychoprophylaxis in Obstetrics (ASPO). This nurse has a private practice and prepares expectant mothers for childbirth, teaches Lamaze method of childbirth, and is well equipped to counsel and teach about pregnancy.

Betty continued her allergy hyposensitization treatment for two years, at which time the therapy regimen was completed. She visited the nurse in ASPO for counseling and delivered successfully via Lamaze.

Case Studies

The names of clients were changed for confidentiality. In almost every case, the clients and their families seemed pleased with the care provided and paid the fees without hesitation. With all nursing care, safety was a first consideration. Self-study, consulting with others, and continuing education enabled provision of quality care to meet clients' needs. Emotional support was provided to the client or family, as required. Communities have a need for these kinds of services; nurses can and should provide this care.

Clients were informed beforehand that their insurance companies may pay for most of the equipment but not for the nursing services. They were also told the fee for the care in advance. Clients wanted this care nonetheless.

Joan Hall, the woman with the T-Tube irrigation, submitted her bill for nursing care to her insurance company and received 80 percent payment. Her company paid 100 percent of the cost for materials. This is an isolated payment by an insurance company for nursing care. However, there should be legislation to mandate all health insurance carriers to provide payment for nursing care, on a fee-for-service basis.

SUMMARY

The sophistication and autonomy that is gained from private practice and the nursing services that it can provide clients may motivate nurses to care for their clients in this way. Greater job satisfaction, improved client care, and greater amounts of time spent with clients and families can be some of the rewards. Teaching clients and families and increased responsibilities in the provision of actual care as new roles are accepted by nurses are also rewarding. Alford and Jensen noted . . . private nurse practitioners will find that they are often the first health professional clients may encounter. Private practitioners assess clients' health status via history taking or physical exam. In some instances, private nurse practitioners include Pap smears, urinalysis, hemoccults, complete blood counts, multiple blood chemistries, other blood profiles, and cultures when screening clients. Often common chronic health problems such as obesity and hypertension are managed by nurses in private practice.

The fact that home visits are made leads people to think that private practice is a home health agency, which it is not.[8]

Rosasco asserts that a higher educated society is demanding quality in health care. One focal point is the nurse as a qualified practitioner. Nurses are now providing care once reserved as the physician's responsibility and role. Equipment used by nurses is sophisticated and complex, requiring considerable knowledge of scientific principles as well as technological skills.[9]

Extensive fragmentation exists as to an overall, universal understanding of what a nurse practitioner does. This same fragmentation does not exist with the physician or other health care providers. Nurses tend to make role definitions, titles, and title definitions difficult preoccupations for themselves. This sort of preoccupation takes away from nursing and keeps it and its members from being all that they could be. The material presented in this chapter should clarify some role definitions. This preoccupation needs to end so that nursing can get involved with delivery of care.

Nurse practitioners can be defined as all nurses who practice nursing. The nurses practicing nursing and contemporaneously being nurse practitioners must meet educational requirements. They must be graduates of nursing schools and legally licensed to practice nursing. Special education beyond nursing school is not required to be a nurse practitioner, or to practice nursing; however, continuing education of some sort is a must.

NOTES

1. Betty Pesznecker, R.N., M.S., "Life Change: A Challenge for Nurse Practitioners," *Nurse Practitioner* 1, no. 1 (September-October 1975): 21–24.

2. Arnold Birenbaum, "Home Care—An Alternative to the High Cost of Hospitalization," *Intellect* 107 (July 1978): 53.

3. Harriett Goodspeed, R.N., "The Independent Practitioner—Can It Survive?" *Journal of Psychiatric Nursing and Mental Health Services* 14 (August 1976): 33.

4. Hilary Smith, "What Do Nurses Do in America?" *American Journal of Nursing* 76, no. 2 (February 1976): 279.

5. *Ibid.*, 280.

6. Kathleen Astin Knafl, "How Nurse Practitioner Students Construct Their Role," *Nursing Outlook* 26, no. 10 (October 1978): 650.

7. Sister Callista Roy and Sister Marcia Obloy, "The Practitioner Movement—Toward a Science of Nursing," *American Journal of Nursing* 78, no. 10 (October 1978): 1700.

8. Dolores Marsh Alford and Janet Molly Jensen, "Reflections on Private Practice," *American Journal of Nursing* 76, no. 12 (December 1976): 1966–1967.

9. Louise C. Rosasco, "Of Nursing Practice and Nurse Practitioners," *Nursing Digest* (May-June 1975): 37.

Chapter 6

Professional Relations

ABOUT PUBLIC RELATIONS

Public relations should be designed to build and increase public confidence, support, and understanding in a given organization or concept. This is best done by a well-communicated set of actions, policies, statements, goals, and philosophies. Proper management will enhance public relations, which consists of two-way communication. According to Donovan, hospitals have recently become concerned over public relations. Hospitals have been isolated as a community resource and tended to be separate from their communities. Hospitals are now realizing the need for two-way communication with their community and now are promoting quality public relations.[1]

Nurses, other professional health care providers, and the public need to be educated about nurses in general. Education specifically about private nurse practitioners is needed for these groups. Nurses also have been isolated as a community resource. This should change. Donovan continues, the history of nursing's public relations is nonimpressive. Problems such as ignorance, conflicting views, and disharmony have prohibited and still prohibit well-communicated, quality public relations. Apathy seems to be the largest problem. Nursing's official statements have lacked good public relations.[2]

Private nurse practitioners can carry their message to their community by exploiting the fact that they are educated and know their business. They need to make themselves understood by others and also to understand nursing, nurses, and themselves. Often nurses do not assert themselves due to a lingering fear of reprisal or negative criticism. Statements from nurses, nursing, and private nurse practitioners would be better received if transmitted precisely, knowledgeably, and assertively.

Nursing can learn by observing public relations practiced by industry. Their public relations are designed to reach the public, employees, and others in the same field. Industry's openness, imagination, durability, and willingness to

81

take a stand are characteristics nursing's public relations personnel should consider. Publicity can be used to obtain favorable opinion.

Private nurse practitioners must constantly maintain ethical business and professional practices. These ethical practices need to be underscored throughout your public and professional relations.

Some special interest groups deserve attention. Examples of these are the public, clients, peers, investors, governmental authorities, nursing authorities, competitors, physicians, hospitals, emergency departments, clinics, educational institutions, and the media. Maintain professional and assertive relations with them to ensure their awareness of your knowledge, capabilities, and credibility as a private nurse practitioner. It will be advantageous for you to make them aware of your purpose as a private nurse practitioner and of your practice's goals and philosophy.

Professional relationships with these groups should be reciprocal. Each party should be willing to give and take. Pursue a policy of fairness, honesty, and open communication. This will help to ensure mutually beneficial and lasting relationships.

Objectives of Professional Relations

People's opinions are an important force affecting organizations. Business people recognize this when they speak of good will. Good will means the attitude of clients, colleagues, the community, and other special interest groups toward your practice. Their good will is necessary for the success of your private practice.

Many objectives may be achieved through professional relations. Some objectives you may seek include:

- prestige
- favorable image
- promotion of understanding
- awareness of services
- good will of special-interest groups
- good will of constituents
- overcoming of false assumptions, misconceptions, or prejudices
- eliminating accusations
- gaining peer group support
- educating the public
- educating peer group
- formulating goals, policies, and purposes
- stimulating public response
- reducing threats

- promoting change
- promoting the practice as a community resource
- promoting referrals

Challenges of Professional Relations

Several areas of challenge to professional relations can aid you in providing care for your clients. Some of them are:

- staying abreast of current events and practices in the profession and being flexible intellectually and in other ways
- listening to your clients
- constantly being aware of the importance and having pride in the quality of your services
- being capable of expressing to others the credibility of yourself and your private practice
- being able to effectively educate others about your role and showing how you can meet their needs
- practicing your profession ethically

To further aid or challenge your practice, you may wish to keep in mind some of the following extrapolations from the consumer relations code. The codes listed here are derived from the 10-point consumer relations code promulgated by the Chamber of Commerce of the United States. They are arranged to apply to a private nursing practice.

1. Protect the health and safety of clients in the provision of services.
2. Utilize advanced technology to meet the highest standards of care at the lowest reasonable fee.
3. Seek out informed views of clients and other groups to help assure their satisfaction from the earliest stages of practice.
4. Simplify, clarify, and honor your services.
5. Maximize the quality of services and encourage fair fee schedules.
6. Eliminate frauds and deceptions; set a goal of honesty in business practices.
7. Be capable of services rendered.
8. Provide clients with information and services either by yourself or by referral.
9. Provide effective channels of communication for receiving and acting on complaints and suggestions from clients or other special interest groups. Utilize the resources of appropriate associations as needed.[3]

Communicating Professional Relations

Successful communication of your private practice's credibility, services, goals, philosophy, and professional relations objectives to the community requires serious time, preparation, and effort. Effective communication takes many forms. Communication is closely tied with the techniques for promoting your practice; these techniques are discussed in depth in Chapter 8, "Promoting the Practice." As you promote your practice, you communicate your professional relations. The meaning of the word promotion covers the area between advertising and publicity and includes both in its application.

PROFESSIONAL RELATIONSHIPS—NEW ROLES

Stanley queries how a nurse practitioner's being a colleague of physicians will affect professional relations. This change requires development of new communication methods with physicians. You may spend a great deal of time with a client and need to make the physician understand your concerns. You have to be assertive, assume responsibility and back up your observations . . . nurse practitioners are on thin ice, they have to learn new skills, develop confidence, and establish positive and new relationships with physicians and clients.[4]

Nurses should begin to explore how they feel about themselves and their interactions with others (whether or not they are professionally related). As a group, nurses could benefit by being more assertive and decisive. Donnelly asks nurses how they feel about themselves. Do you like your behavior at work and do you freely express yourself? Do you carry out unreasonable work requests and drop everything for the physician? Are you able to ventilate your feelings at the moment you feel them? Do you apply for a promotion or do you hint about it? If some of these problems are yours, you need to change. You can break these patterns by becoming more assertive; then you will be a more relaxed, efficient, fulfilled person and nurse.[5]

When you become more assertive, your professional relations will rise to meaningful levels. Others will recognize the credibility of your private practice. Others will like you more, and you will be happier. Rodin claims that the image of nursing is not realistic. The nurses' career possibilities are limited only by their imaginations, amount of continuing education, and aggressiveness. Nurses have let themselves be conditioned to a handmaiden role. Nursing needs to work for a collaborative role with physicians. This may enlighten nurses and physicians to the full potential of the nurse. Neither nursing nor medicine alone has all the answers, we must work together.[6]

Learning how to say NO is very important also. You should develop this capability since there will be times you will have to say NO! You may have to decline from providing a service whether it be requested from a client or physician. When you cannot provide the care requested, but would like to, the best answer is NO. Offer your assistance by trying to locate a qualified provider of the requested service.

Realizing how and when to say no is difficult, says Close. Think of a time when someone asked you to do something you didn't want to do. You just couldn't say no and ended up regretting it. Two kinds of people it's hard to say no to are people you feel sorry for and people you care for. Learn to say no tactfully and remember that you can always say yes. Saying yes and no can enable you to become more comfortable in relationships.[7]

Being more assertive and expressive will enable you to be a happier and safer nurse practitioner. What nurse can always say yes? To always say yes is unrealistic. Nurses, especially those entering private practice, should begin to develop these attributes.

Nurse-Physician Collaboration

Keeping channels of communication open with the client's physician is of extreme importance. The physician must be provided with feedback from you about the progress of the client. When communicating with the physician, you will be provided with new orders as the medical regimen changes. This is the time to inform the physician of changes in the client's nursing regimen.

In keeping the physician informed, you will be binding your relationship. The physician will learn to trust you more and will refer clients to you more frequently. Some may invite you to their practices to explain techniques of care for a client that they may have in mind for future referral to your practice.

Donovan states that hospital administrators, physicians, public opinion molders, and the public take nurses for granted. The remedy lies in educating physicians and others about nurses' capabilities. The public does not understand the nursing problem. This problem, as Donovan states, is the conflict between the traditional role of the nurse and the need for increased professional status and adequate remuneration.[8]

Entering private practice is a break from the traditional role. Increased collaboration with physicians and accepting new roles is increasing professional status; the adequate remuneration will follow.

Many physicians do not like quality of care questions from nurses. Some physicians perceive them as interference with medical practice or as an infringement upon their professional prerogatives, says Hershey. Nurses raising such questions run the risks of uncomfortable relationships, threats of retaliation, loss of cooperation, collaboration or referrals. Physicians have a responsibility to cooperate and collaborate with nurses.[9]

Some physicians do not like questions from nurses. Your questions are a legitimate and professional function. You should ask questions, however, remain tactful and polite when doing so. If there is no response, continue to ask the question again, remaining assertive and firm. Scheduling an appointment for collaboration with the physician may prove beneficial in alleviating physician anxiety.

Schrader believes that nurses used to be taught in nursing schools to use indirect communication with physicians. In the last several years nurses have used nursing diagnosis, observations, and conclusions to enable their communication with physicians to be strengthened and more direct. Indirect dialogue perpetuates the nurse's subordinate role to physicians. Nurses wishing to be recognized as professional colleagues to physicians, should stop the doctor-nurse game.[10]

Most physicians will accept your queries and respond to them. Asking questions of physicians is a way of beginning collaboration. The physician who answers your question or explains a point of view feels needed and may begin to comprehend his or her role regarding a private nursing practice. The Physician's Questionnaire, Exhibit 4-1, can be used as a method of developing professional relationships with physicians. This can go a long way in developing future interaction. Often the client's physician will ask you questions. Once this occurs, there is positive collaboration for the betterment of client care.

Relationships with Clients and Families

Relating with your clients and their families provides them with the trust and confidence they need in you as a professional providing their health care. Family interaction is prohibitive when the client has no family, when they cannot be reached, or when the client wants the care held in confidence. Bring the family into the picture when needed or when the client wants them to be included. Use good judgment and tact in your communication. If needed, consult with another nurse or the physician for advice about the care you will provide or for advice about interaction with the client or family.

Illness is often more evident in verbal behavior than in actions. Talking with your clients is an important aspect of your constructive nursing intervention. Simple, clear guidelines encourage verbal exchanges between nurses and clients. As professionals, nurses ought to have a wide range of interpersonal procedures available for their recall, to use as the work situation requires.

Verbal communication is one of the nurse's primary tools for meeting the client's emotional needs. This leads to a professional, constructive, and therapeutic relationship between the nurse and client. Ill persons have emotional needs; they may be anxious, fearful, angry, depressed, or disturbed. Emotional problems are not confined to a psychiatric hospital; you will run into them in your clients in your practice.

Many clients in hospitals have a psychiatric problem contemporaneously with a physical problem. People will come to your practice, as they do to a hospital, for treatment of a physical problem. Later, through interactions, nurses discover and treat the emotional or psychiatric needs. Nurses need to care for the whole person and not just the physical needs. These needs exist in the client and the family. Your interaction with those involved with the client is needed, to help everyone through a hardship.

A tool for reducing tension and anxiety is ventilation, which means talking about your feelings. There must be a good listener present; that is you, the nurse. Nurses sometimes avoid clients' and families' questions and requests to talk, because they don't know how to interact as well as they could.

Nurses can realize a great opportunity to provide therapy in ways other than hands on. They can develop their communication skills, be good listeners, and encourage the client or family to cope with their current situation. Nurses should welcome this increased responsibility, because they are interested in promoting health, but few have been prepared for it adequately. Hays and Larson say the nurse's role is to provide the client with the opportunity: (1) to identify and explore problems in relating to others, (2) to discover healthy ways of meeting emotional needs, and (3) to experience a satisfying interpersonal relationship.[11]

As the nurse you must make your role clear; this enables communication to flow freely. Be aware that what you say to your clients or within their hearing to others can be evaluated as therapeutic or harmful. Be sure others understand your role. Stanley sees the nurse practitioner as a new concept in health care. Many clients will not understand the difference between the nurse practitioner and the physician. Tell them you are a nurse practitioner and what your role is. Many clients will say 'Thank you, Doctor,' anyhow. Clients have accepted nurse practitioners well because once they see you, they will usually be comfortable seeing you again.[12]

Some techniques to promote communication include using a quiet area so that you and whomever you are talking with can hear one another; this would also allow for confidentiality. When the family or client becomes anxious, the topic should be changed. Face one another, speak loudly, clearly, slowly, and have enough light so you can see one another's faces.

Make yourself available to the family or client for talk. Observing that there is a need to talk, offer comments to the family or client letting them know that they can begin. Encourage them to continue talking, while you listen.

Focus the client or family on an area that needs more discussion. Direct the conversation to a special area for you or the client to give information. There are many texts on communication, in the event you need strengthening in this area. If the client or family member has an emotional outburst, it is best for you to remain calm; he or she will usually emulate your calm.

Your first visit with the client and family is vital to your success as a promoter of their health. This initial visit is when they decide if you are going to be helpful, if they like you, if they want to let you touch the client, if you can come into their home, and if they will call upon you again. Verbal communication is the key. Also, it is important to touch your clients to let them realize that you have empathy and feeling for them as individuals and do not think of them as just another client.

The first visit is when you develop your client's history by being a good listener and asking appropriate questions. The family could be present to observe your nursing care. Let them and the client see you wash your hands before checking vital signs. Let them see that you are able to touch the client to develop trust. The family, client, and you will probably be nervous; by communicating and touching, you can take control and perform care well. Once care begins, it may be best to have the family leave you with your client. Use judgment because often a spouse will want to stay, or the client may insist on having others there.

The client and family should be included in the client's care. Far too often clients are left lying in beds unable to care for themselves simply because no one said they could, or taught them how to, help themselves.

Rodin claims clients should be able to take part in their own care. Too often they are left in bed feeling like an object at everyone's mercy. Strive to include clients in planning for their return to daily life.[13]

In building an accepting, supporting, and trusting relationship with the client and family, consider that you will leave them one day to function on their own. You may have to wean them from your care. Try not to develop a dependency relationship; help clients and families to function on their own.

A nurse who builds an accepting, supporting, and trusting relationship with clients can avoid a dependency relationship to allow the client and family to function on their own. There are two ways this may be done. First, the nurse should adhere to a firm professional attitude, maintaining professional conduct. Second, the nurse should reward or praise the client for gaining insight into self-care. The nurse in behaving in these ways will aid the client and family to function independently, Reinhardt and Quinn assert.[14]

Collaboration with Nurses

Nurses should communicate openly among themselves, thereby enhancing nursing and nursing care. Nurses need to refer clients to one another more frequently than they do now. For some unknown reason, nurses are reluctant to do this. They often feel it is illegal to do so, that this referral to another nurse would be using the client or admitting a personal defeat or incompetency. It is not any of these things. It would be practicing better nursing care.

Communication with other nurses or referring clients to other nurses enhances our profession in the public's eye as well as in the eyes of the professions. This communication could bring clients to you, as well as allow your referral to other nurses. Communication allows nurses to get together to discuss care plans for clients. Nurses need to openly share with other nurses on an informal basis as physicians do. Having more than one private nursing practice in your community would enhance clients' health care.

Meet with other nurses for consultation, collaboration, or question sessions in order to insure open and ongoing communication. Becoming a member of various nursing organizations or associations can be helpful for collaboration with other nurses. Also, you will hear of current events in the profession. Meeting with other nurses or becoming a member of professional associations will develop your professional relations greatly.

Complaints

Complaints must be expected in even the best run organizations. They are unpleasant. Proper handling of complaints can be a valuable device for maintaining client relations. Some principles that may be useful are:

- Be prompt; tardiness aggravates the client.
- Be specific; show your client that you understand the complaint and are not putting him or her off.
- Be polite.
- Be honest.
- Be ethical.
- Be firm.
- Listen to your client.
- Explain your point of view.
- Resolve the complaint with fairness to the client and you.

Physician's Assistant—An Alternative Plan

Physician Assistant or Physician Associate (PA) programs rely heavily on their affiliated clinical campus of physicians' offices for their education. They take classroom instruction and make use of community clinics, depending on the needs of the program. Their training is coordinated to provide a combination of ambulatory and in-patient care, plus private practice in primary care.

The private practice in primary care is what nursing education is lacking and sorely needs.

Physicians in private practice function as preceptors for actual clinical training. The clinical setting is the physician's office. Therefore the PAs seem to be in line for entry into private practice. It is easy for the nursing profession to relax, sit back, and let them provide the kinds of care to America's public that the nursing profession should provide, and this may happen.

But, there are many difficulties with PA programs and their graduates. First, some of the programs have already closed. Second, the PAs are finding it extremely difficult to obtain employment. They have not got the upward mobility that nurses have. Various states have vague laws governing their roles, and usually they must work directly under the supervision of a hiring physician. They are not as free as the nurse to enter private practice. Nurses fail to realize what a good position they are in. They should exercise this privilege before they lose it.

Some other difficulties for PAs are that there are no licensure requirements for them in many states. They are held in a state of limbo. Nurses often refuse to accept orders from PAs, as they would accept orders from physicians.

Since many of the original schools closed, there are fewer and fewer PA graduates each year. It is difficult to predict the future of the PA, but many physicians have expressed concern that the PA may turn into a substitute physician, something the medical profession does not want.

The role and function of PAs in America's health care system needs clarification; nursing needs this, too, but not as much as the PAs. Nursing is viable and solidly entrenched with the public, government, and medical profession. Nurses could make use of this strong position and take the roles of private practice like true professionals.

Nurses' Questions

Since the media have had increasing numbers of articles on private nursing practice, the author has received many questionnaires from interested nurses. Some of these nurses were simply curious, and others were genuinely interested in developing their own practice. You may receive questionnaires as your practice develops. Or, you may wish to send a questionnaire to a private nurse practitioner, to provide you with further data for development of your practice, or to decide whether to enter private practice.

Table 6-1 contains several questions nurses often ask. These questions can be used during consultation with private nurse practitioners or for mailing to private nurse practitioners. It is a good idea to send a self-addressed, stamped envelope with the questionnaire, as a courtesy. This questionnaire can be a means of opening a professional relationship with other private nurse practitioners.

Competition

Why open a private practice when you would be competing with existing health care providers? Will stepping on their toes make it more difficult for nurses in general? Competition is healthy, and the American system of free enterprise allows it. Other health care providers should welcome your practice.

It may sound strange to talk of private nursing practice as a business, because it is a new concept for us to get used to. Physicians are quite familiar with their practices as businesses and compete with one another all the time, and yet there is no antagonism between them; they support one another and refer to one another. They also refer to other health care providers who have private practices.

Physicians are businessmen; they have two functions contemporaneously, and no one questions their legal and moral ethics. The same trust and status easily can be granted to the nurse in private practice. The public's trust in receiving health care by nurses from private practice could be gained quickly by associating with physicians' practices. Promoting good professional relations will win the status nurses deserve.

Competition with Physicians

Physicians can be your primary source of referral. They are quick to understand the private practice concept in total. Many physicians will like it and understand how it can benefit clients. Often physicians will offer more support than nurses.

The physicians in my community were not afraid of losing their business. They knew that we would care for the same clients, and they knew that a nursing practice would help the client. Physicians often understand the business world and competition more than nurses do because they deal with it daily. Many physicians respect anything that will provide more and better health care to clients.

One thing that impressed me while consulting with physicians was how very dedicated to medicine and to their clients they are. In the years before opening private practice, I felt physicians were in business to earn a great deal of money. By making friends with some physicians, I learned that they want to earn their just reward (and this is respectable), but that they do care genuinely about their clients.

Physicians also cared for me; they referred clients, trusted, taught, aided, and advised me when needed. Often, the public and nurses are quick to

Table 6-1 Private Nurse Practitioner Questionnaire

Group A: General Data

1. How long has your practice been operational?
2. What title do you attribute to yourself while practicing as a private nurse practitioner?
3. What title do you feel nurse practitioners should use?
4. What title is utilized for your staff?
5. What is your definition of a private nurse practitioner?
6. What are the attitudes towards you from these sources?
   a. American Medical Society
   b. American Nurses Association
   c. various local nursing associations
   d. local medical society
   e. nursing peers
   f. local nurses
   g. local physicians
   h. local community
   i. local nursing schools
   j. local hospitals
   k. Public Health Department
   l. visiting nurses associations
   m. Health Department
   n. Education Department
   o. local clinics
7. What are your future plans for your practice?
8. Describe the future of private nursing practice as you see it.

Group B: Management of Private Practice

1. Are you independent or interdependent in working with other local health care providers and agencies?
2. What professional disciplines does your staff comprise?
3. What is your total number of staff and in which disciplines?
4. How many hours per week, month, or year are devoted to:
   a. home visits
   b. office visits
   c. other
5. What percent of the total number of client visits do each of the following hold?
   a. home visits

b. office visits
c. other
6. Is malpractice insurance a prerequisite to conducting a private nursing practice in your locale?
7. Do you have malpractice insurance?
8. Explain your malpractice insurance, if you have it.
9. What legal advice did you find necessary for entrance into private practice?
10. Do you receive complaints?
11. What complaint is most frequent?
12. How do you handle complaints?
13. Are you the sole owner, or do you have a partner?
14. Include a copy of your goals and philosophy.
15. What difficulties were encountered?
16. What was the largest difficulty?
17. How did you work them out?
18. Is your practice located in your home, rented building, or other location?

Group C: Preparation for Private Practice

1. What preparation do you feel is needed by nurses to enter private practice?
2. What is or was your preparation for private practice?
   a. education—to what extent?
      • generic
      • continuing education
   b. experience—to what extent?
   c. other
3. What preparation is required in your locale?

Group D: Client Data

1. What is your client census per week, month, and year?
2. How much time is spent with clients?
3. What percentage of clients request and receive:
   a. home visits
   b. office visits
   c. other
4. What are the income ranges of your clients?
5. What age groups are your clients?
6. Which age groups request the most and least of your services?
7. What types of services are requested by each age group?
8. List the number of clients your practice had for each six months from its inception to the present.

9. Are your clients satisfied with your services?
10. Do clients accept you as their health provider?

Group E: Promotion of Private Practice

1. How do you inform community members of your practice and services?
2. Do you advertise? If so, where?
3. What are your referral sources?

Group F: Services and Fees

1. Include a copy of your schedule of nursing services.
2. Include a copy of your fee schedule.
3. How do you determine fees?
   a. by time
   b. by responsibility
   c. by type of care
   d. by distance traveled
   e. other
4. What type of care is primarily requested?

Group G: Finances

1. What is the primary mechanism used by your clients to reimburse you for services?
2. What and how do you pay staff?
3. What were your start-up costs?
4. How did you fund these start-up costs?
5. What are your monthly expenses?
6. Is the financial status of your practice improving?

Group H: Community

1. Describe your community:
   a. urban
   b. suburban
   c. rural
   d. other
2. What is the availability of health care in your community?
3. How did you assess your community?

Group I: Personal

1. Why did you enter private practice?
2. Is traditional employment necessary while in private practice?
3. If holding traditional employment, what is it?
4. What specialties are you skilled in?
5. What is your age?
6. What percentage of your total income is from your practice?

Please include any necessary data that may have been overlooked by this questionnaire.

---

criticize physicians; seldom do we hear praise for them. Developing relationships with physicians should enable you to respect and understand them more.

The physician in your community may be the last person for you to worry about unless you practice illegally. If you practice illegally and jeopardize client care, the physician will probably be the first to correct the situation. Most physicians care about the public's welfare.

Physicians probably have practices in every town in America. Some towns have more than one of the same type. This situation should produce no problem, if the need is there. Therefore, the competition with physicians should not be threatening or devastating to either of you.

Beason says some physicians may fear financial competition. Nurses argue that physicians are only concerned about crowding the health care field. It is unlikely that nurses would compete directly with physicians, since nurses provide care that physicians have bypassed. There may be a competition question when nurses provide care in overlapping areas.[15]

Competition With Private Nurse Practitioners

Nurses often worry about each other and frequently criticize one another too quickly. The time has come for a uniform national effort on every nurse's part to strengthen the profession and not to tear it apart.

Professional jealousy and the energy that goes into it could be better spent delivering client care. When more than one private nursing practice appears in the same town, the practices should work together, support one another, refer to each other, and encourage other nurses to open private practices.

The existence of competition raises public awareness of nursing practices. An increased number of private practices will yield more health care delivery. The public could begin to conceptualize the value in care provided through nursing practices. Several practices, some general and some specialized, may serve a town; they will probably greatly enhance the community's health care system.

A second nursing practice opened in my community about one year after I established my practice. My partner went into private practice for herself. Client referral and consultation between the private nurse practitioners aided each practice greatly. Actually, no competition existed because of the great need for more health care in our community.

Referrals

The nursing practice is advised to service a radius of 15 to 20 miles at the most. Letters of introduction, business cards, and a list of services can be sent to physicians in the 15- to 20-mile radius. These contacts are particularly helpful if the physician's specialty is similar to the nursing services you offer. Some general practitioners may have clients who need the type of nursing care your practice offers.

Hospitals, local Public Health Departments, clinics, and other nurses also could be mailed this material. From these sources would come referrals for nursing care provided by your practice. Geyman et al. relate that referrals and consultations are a vital method to ensure and provide clients with the most desirable quality of care. Referrals represent an important way to provide continuing education to physicians regarding the sharing of client-care responsibility.[16]

Randolph explained that her client load ranged from 2 to 20 clients at a time. Most of her referrals came from physicians, but some came from the local school system, clients themselves, the phone book, clergy, and various community organizations. Her work load varied often with little control; in a week, she said, you could lose almost half a client load. In the summer, referrals were slow because people were on vacation.[17]

Membership in nursing associations, besides allowing collaboration with nurses, is a good way to let other nurses know of your practice. Hopefully, these associations or members will refer clients when appropriate.

First Client

My first client was a young lady, age 9, who visited the practice with her mother. The client's mother had read about the practice in a local newspaper story. This client received injections for allergy care (hyposensitization) as ordered and strictly outlined by her allergist. They came to the private nursing practice because the cost for care was lower, and the practice was close to home.

This marked the beginning of my practice: an actual client came for hypo-sensitization injections by a nurse. Physician's orders were followed, and the client's mother paid the fee after each visit. The first client was about 6 months in coming and came for 2 years, until her regimen was completed.

Randolph said that even after three years, her nursing practice did not have a full complement of clients. She found that there is an initiation rite for people in private practice; they must wait and work long periods of time establishing their practice and earning a name in the community. She was accepted as a professional by other professionals; then she had to get the acceptance of clients. Her first client came for physician's care, but Randolph developed a positive relationship with this client and treated her for over a year. Later, the first client referred her son for care.[18]

SUMMARY

As physicians discontinue making home visits and other services, nurses will start filling these needs. Making your community aware that you can meet some of their health care needs is the key to success.

Proper professional relations will enhance your private nursing practice. Successful professional relations will stimulate community awareness, community usage, referrals, acceptance, status, and development of your private practice. It will also eliminate confusion regarding what your practice does and will help eliminate complaints. Physician and client acceptance will be heightened through the effective use of quality professional relations.

Your clients may even be more satisfied with care from your nursing practice. Lewis and Cheyovich asserted that clients who received care from nurse practitioners were more satisfied with their care than those clients who did not receive care from nurse practitioners. The costs of care were lower as clients were not hospitalized as frequently. There was no problem with clients accepting the nurse practitioners.[19]

It has been demonstrated that clients are more satisfied with care from family nurse practitioners than from traditional care providers. Physicians, Linn says, are included in these traditional care providers. Clients evaluated nurse practitioners more favorably than traditional nurses. In the eyes of the client, the nurse practitioner is an effective new source of health care.[20]

NOTES

1. Helen M. Donovan, *Nursing Service Administration Managing the Enterprise* (Saint Louis: The C. V. Mosby Company, 1975), p. 244.

2. *Ibid.,* p. 246.

3. Philip Lesly, ed., *Lesly's Public Relations Handbook* (Englewood Cliffs, N.J.: Prentice-Hall, Inc., 1971), p, 173.

4. Linda Stanley, R.N., B.S.N., " 'Expanded-Role' Nursing Hits the Hospitals," *RN* 41, no. 10 (October 1978): 57–59.

5. Gloria Ferraro Donnelly, R.N., M.S.N., "How to Soothe a Savage Surgeon," *RN* 41, no. 11 (November 1978): 45.

6. Rita Rodin, "Today's Florence Nightingales Everything's Changed but the Idealism," *Working Woman* 3 (May 1978): 31–35.

7. Henry T. Close, "On Saying NO to People: A Pastoral Letter," *Journal of Nursing Digest* 3 (January-February 1975): 49, 52.

8. Helen M. Donovan, *Nursing Service Administration Managing the Enterprise* (Saint Louis: The C.V. Mosby Company, 1975), p. 245.

9. Nathan Hershey, "Physician Reaction to Quality of Care Assessment by Nurses," *The Hospital Medical Staff* 5, no. 7 (July 1976): 10.

10. Elinor Schrader, ed., "Can Nurses Communicate Directly With Physicians?" *AORN Journal* 28, no. 2 (August 1978): 193–4.

11. Joyce Hays, R.N. and Kenneth Larson, R.N., *Interacting With Patients* (New York: Macmillan Co., 1963), p. 2.

12. Linda Stanley, R.N., B.S.N., " 'Expanded-Role' Nursing Hits the Hospitals," *RN* 41, no. 10 (October 1978): 58.

13. Rita Rodin, "Today's Florence Nightingales—Everything's Changed but the Idealism," *Working Woman* 3 (May 1978): 32.

14. Adina M. Reinhardt and Mildred D. Quinn, *Family-Centered Community Nursing* (Saint Louis: The C. V. Mosby Company, 1978), p. 140.

15. Cathy Beason, ed., "Nurse Practitioners: The Flak From Doctors is Getting Heavier," *RN* 41, no. 10 (October 1978): 36.

16. John P. Geyman, M.D., Thomas C. Brown, Ph.D., and Kevin Rivers, A.B., "Referrals in Family Practice: A Comparative Study by Geographic Region and Practice Setting," *The Journal of Family Practice* 3, no. 2 (April 1976): 167.

17. Gretchen T. Randolph, "Experiences in Private Practice," *Journal of Psychiatric Nursing* 13 (November-December 1975): 18.

18. *Ibid.*, p. 17.

19. Charles E. Lewis, M.D., Sc.D. and Therese K. Cheyovich, R.N., M.S., "Who is a Nurse Practitioner? Processes of Care and Patients' and Physicians' Perceptions," *Medical Care* 14, no. 4 (April 1976): 367.

20. Lawrence S. Linn, Ph.D., "Patient Acceptance of the Family Nurse Practitioner," *Medical Care* 14, no. 4 (April 1976): 363.

Chapter 7

The Professional Corporation

PREPARING FOR A PROFESSIONAL CORPORATION

Familiarization with business corporate laws regarding professional service corporations is needed to enable you to decide whether to create a professional corporation (PC). Deciding whether to form a PC can be difficult. An attorney and an accountant should be consulted prior to forming one. These sources and this chapter will aid you in understanding the pros and cons of a PC related to your private practice and you. Several necessities should be considered prior to forming a PC.

- Decide who will be the professional corporation's:
  a. president
  b. treasurer
  c. secretary
- Keep minutes—initial and ongoing.
- Decide the corporate name.
- Determine costs of corporating.
- Determine costs of dissolution.
- Determine maintenance costs.
- Get an estimate of attorney and accountant fees.
- List the advantages of PC.
- List the disadvantages of PC.
- Find out what forms are needed.
- Familiarize yourself with the laws governing PCs.
- Find out about stocks and stockholders.
- Investigate liability insurance for you and the PC.

Generally, recognized professions allowed to form PCs are:

- architects
- chiropractors
- dentists
- dental hygienists
- engineers
- surveyors
- masseurs and masseuses
- nurses (professional, licensed, vocational)
- ophthalmic dispensers
- optometrists
- osteopathic physicians
- pharmacists
- physicians
- physiotherapists
- podiatrists
- psychologists (certified)
- veterinarians
- public accountants (certified)
- shorthand reporters (certified)
- social workers (certified)

These professions are restricted to performing only the practice indicated by their title. Request a copy of the business corporate laws from your governing capital.

President/Treasurer/Secretary

Corporations and PCs require officers; usually they are limited to three. Whoever actually owns the private nursing practice should be the president. A spouse, relative, or friend could hold the office of treasurer or secretary.

Minutes

Initially, minutes have to be kept to demonstrate official corporate action. It is in these minutes that the officers and stockholders will be mentioned. Ongoing minutes are necessary as mandated by law.

Corporation Title

There can be a great deal of benefit in the firm name. A continuing name can be valuable and deserves attention. According to Burke and Zaloom, these questions require strong consideration:

1. Does your governing body allow your PC to hold the name of the current partnership, including retired or deceased partners?
2. Does the corporate name have to change if a partner whose name is in the corporate name dies, retires, or withdraws?
3. What are the restrictions limiting the descriptive wording of the name?
4. Is appendage wording mandated?
5. What is the cost to change the name?
6. Are there conflicts between these answers and professional ethics? If so, what are they?[1]

The name may contain only words that could describe the profession the corporation is authorized to practice. The effect of this provision is to prohibit the inclusion in the name of a professional service corporation the words incorporated or limited (and their abbreviations Inc. and Ltd.) and to prohibit the use of assumed names by professional service corporations formed to practice any profession. The corporate name must end with the words Professional Corporation or the abbreviation PC. Some governing agencies may allow you to establish incorporations or limiteds.

Choosing a name that speaks for itself will convey your services to your public. The governing agency will probably check your requested title against others similar to it. If your desired name is already being used, or is close to one already in use, you will have to choose another name. This rule eliminates public ambiguity.

Professional Corporation Costs

To form a PC, a large start-up fee is charged. It is larger than maintenance fees and may be prohibitive. The fee for forming my PC was $650, a one-time fee. Maintaining fees for the PC (paid to the governing agency) were $125 annually. Lawyers and accountants who aid you in filing corporate forms quarterly and annually also charge.

McShane and Smith established a private practice in 1978. Their name is Person to Person, Inc. Their cost of incorporation, rather than professionally corporating, was $450.[2]

In the event that you wish to dissolve your corporate status, you must pay a dissolution fee. I chose to go through a corporate dissolution after having a PC for one year. The decision for this was based on high costs and amounts of work involved with maintaining the PC. Dissolution costs were $225. There was no prerequisite for me to form a PC for entry into private practice. The reason for forming the professional corporation was to demonstrate professionalism.

Advantages

According to Agree, tax benefits are derived from private practice. These tax benefits can help you through financially difficult years. One private practitioner noted that during the first years of private practice business expenses and losses were offset by tax returns from traditional employment, enabling this private practitioner to break even. Tax deductions for private practice range from rent and telephone to automobile and insurance.[3]

You may be able to put a great percentage of your income into pension funds or profit sharing. These investments are not taxed until the funds are terminated.

Forming a PC has the advantage of denoting professionalism. In some areas, incorporating may protect your homes and families from malpractice suits, because the liability stops at the corporation. This safeguard does not hold true for all areas; it can be determined from your governing agency.

McShane and Smith found that incorporating protected their homes and families from malpractice suits. The liability did stop at their corporation.[4]

Disadvantages

The costs of establishing and maintaining a PC are the most prominent disadvantages to forming one. These costs may prove to be unnecessary, so it is important to explore the full impact of a PC on your practice in your area. Time and energy are involved in establishing and maintaining a PC. Establishment can take months, and it can be tiring.

Stockholders, usually only yourself and at times the other officers, have to hold regular meetings and prepare appropriate minutes. This record keeping can absorb a great deal of time.

The formation of a PC usually does not provide the professional nurse with the security of an assumed name. McShane and Smith were afforded this security only because they formed an incorporation rather than a professional corporation. The legal difference lies in the fact that an assumed name means that in the event of being sued, the corporation name is sued. You, the individual, cannot be sued; you are an employee of that corporation.

In my area of practice, the owner-president of the PC is held accountable for its actions. Nonprofessionals are mandated to form limiteds (Ltd.) and incorporations (Inc.) rather than professional corporations. PCs are reserved for the professionals. Thus the individual professionals are held accountable for their behavior. Nonprofessionals, such as auto mechanics who own a garage or gas station, would have to establish an Inc. or Ltd. This person cannot be personally sued or held liable for negligent acts related to the corporation services.

Whether your laws provide you with security behind an assumed name, you and any type of corporation, even if you own it, are two separate entities. Since a corporation and its owner are two separate entities, it may be wise to consider malpractice insurance for yourself and for the corporation. This duplication of costs can be prohibitive to forming a PC.

Often, completion of specialized forms is required by the regulatory agency. These forms are lengthy, confusing, and frequently require the aid of an attorney and accountant. These forms must be submitted to the regulatory agency as prescribed—quarterly, semiannually, or annually—as a professional responsibility of a PC.

The disadvantages of a PC may dissuade you from establishing one. Be certain, however, to ascertain whether a PC is a prerequisite to private practice in your area.

Establishing Legality

The attorneys in the regulatory agency of my area took eight months to recognize that nurses could form PCs, even though nurses were included in the business corporate laws as professionals. At the time, only physicians had been forming PCs. Our PC was the first established by a nurse in the corporate area. I chose a corporate name that denotes the geographic area my private practice services—Professional Nursing of Long Island.

At the onset of the first year of private practice, the Secretary of the New York State Board of Examiners of Nurses responded to my request to establish legality for nurses in this state to enter into private practice. The Secretary refers to the practice as a storefront and independent practice which it was so often called in the beginning. Storefront and independent are misnomers used by several nurses. The letter read:

> This letter responds to yours in which you described the services you propose to offer in a storefront that would sell fee-for-nursing service.
>
> I have discussed your letter with members of the Department, including legal counsel. We are advised by legal counsel that your proposal to engage in independent nursing practice is legal. Such independent nursing practice must fall within the definition of nurs-

ing contained in Chapter 987 of the laws of 1971, Title VIII, Article 139, Section 6901. This new law, which was signed by Governor Rockefeller on July 2, becomes effective September 1, 1971. The definition is as follows:

'The practice of the profession of nursing as a registered professional nurse is defined as performing service in the maintenance of health, prevention of illness and care of the sick requiring the application of principles of nursing based on biological, physical and social sciences such as supervising and providing nursing care and treatment through observation of a patient's condition, recording such observations, applying appropriate nursing measures, and executing orders concerning treatment and medication issued by a licensed or otherwise legally authorized physician or dentist.

'The practice of nursing as a licensed practical nurse is defined as performing assigned duties and acts in the care of the sick under the direction of a registered professional nurse or a licensed or otherwise legally authorized physician or dentist requiring an understanding of nursing but not requiring the professional service as defined in subdivision one.'

One of our concerns is that in a storefront setting there would seem to exist the potential for practicing beyond the legal scope of practice of the profession. You will need to be aware of this and provide a framework for practice to ensure that the nursing service provided in the storefront is within the legal definition of nursing.

Have you considered the possibility of forming a professional service corporation for the purpose of rendering professional services as authorized under Article 15 of the Business Corporation Law? Information concerning professional service corporations is enclosed. You may want to obtain legal advice before considering the desirability of forming a professional service corporation.

Please keep in touch. We will be interested in knowing how your proposal develops.

Sincerely,
Secretary, State Board of
Examiners of Nurses
Division of Professional Education
The State Education Department

SUMMARY

Establishing a PC will definitely show professionalism. A PC may be desirable at the outset of your practice. Later you may dissolve the PC status and retain your name without the PC after it.

Usually you can conduct your practice legally and professionally without the PC, that is, the PC is not usually a prerequisite for nurses going into private practice. It may be wise not to form a PC until your practice is generating substantially high levels of revenue, or until your attorney or accountant advises you to form one.

Tax write-offs or deductions are still available without the PC status; any business can incur losses and expenses. Unless there is security behind an assumed name or forming a PC is a prerequisite to opening a practice, the money that would go for forming a PC may be better spent on another aspect of the private practice.

This assessment should not be too difficult to perform. It is worth some time and effort to assess PCs and how they would affect you and your practice.

NOTES

1. William J. Burke and Basil J. Zaloom, *Blueprint for Professional Service Corporations* (New York: Thomas Y. Crowell Company, 1970), p. 74–5.

2. Nancy Gerberding McShane and Elizabeth McDowell Smith, "Starting a Private Practice in Mental Health Nursing," *American Journal of Nursing* 78, no. 12 (December 1978): 2068–9.

3. Betty C. Agree, "Beginning an Independent Nursing Practice," *American Journal of Nursing* 74 no. 4 (April 1974): 641.

4. Nancy Gerberding McShane and Elizabeth McDowell Smith, "Starting a Private Practice in Mental Health Nursing," *American Journal of Nursing* 78, no. 12 (December 1978): 2069.

Chapter 8

Promoting the Practice

PUBLICITY

Promoting your services and developing public and professional relations go hand in hand; they fall under the broad definition of communications. The function of publicity is to tell your story. Advertising your private practice and how it can help the community enables clients to utilize your practice fully. Satisfied clients transfer their satisfaction to you and your practice. Clients are directly important to the growth of your practice.

According to Petrof, Carusone, and McDavid, advertising and personal selling carry the brunt of publicity for most organizations. Every good business recognizes the value of positive publicity.[1]

Good client relations depend on your knowledge of your market, services, and capabilities. Matching services with client needs produces satisfaction and successful nursing care. These factors are the most important in determining profitability, community image, and personal satisfaction.

Advertising

According to Cook, the goal of advertising should be to develop clients not for a one-time relationship but for ongoing relationships. It is easier to keep an old client than to obtain new ones, although you will lose some clients as they move out of your area or as their health care needs change. New clients are needed to break even financially, particularly if you want your practice to grow.[2]

Advertising has three main functions: to inform, persuade, and remind the public. While you seek new clients by advertising, you can create a favorable image for your practice. Advertising must be directed to an audience; to find the right message, ask yourself what message to give, whom to give it to, where to give it, and when to give it.

Ethical, moral, professional, and legal aspects relate to the nursing profession and to your local ordinances. The agency governing nursing in your area should be contacted for a directive, advice, and aid in your advertising. Advertising, as industry does, may not be ethical, commonplace, and/or legal in your jurisdiction for nursing. Be certain to research the governing codes applicable to you.

Several ethically acceptable techniques for your publicity would be acceptable when applied judiciously.

- friends
- notices of introduction
- business cards
- location of practice
- hanging a shingle
- peer interest
- peer group endorsement
- speaking engagements
- trade journals
- yellow pages
- public service announcements
- interviews

Professional relations with colleagues and consultants can generate sizable numbers of referrals. Keeping your advertising low key but in the public view is a strong, subtle, and appropriate method for raising awareness of your practice and its services. Health care professions are often restricted from hard-sell advertising, which would utilize television, radio, magazine, or newspaper advertisements. Hard-sell publicity may be unethical or in fact undesirable and financially prohibitive.

Friends

Entering private practice will quickly teach you who your real friends are. They are the people who stand by you, support you emotionally, advise, and aid you. They may donate equipment, time, services, or funds, and they will have faith and understanding in your business venture.

Even friends who are not nurses will carry information to others regarding your practice. They may help educate community members about private nursing practices. Their trust in you will be transmitted to those with whom they talk. Friends will help your practice to become more established.

Introductions

The Physician's Questionnaire, Exhibit 4-1, is a professionally acceptable method of informing colleagues of your services. Notices of introduction and business cards, sent to colleagues and significant agencies (health care or others), generate awareness and referrals to your practice.

Printing costs vary, but they are not prohibitive. Notices of introduction and business cards can be mailed or delivered personally; either way, they are useful. Always carry business cards with you so that you can provide them to others as needed.

Table 6-1, Private Nurse Practitioner Questionnaire, shows a method of introducing yourself to other nurses. Exhibits 8-1 and 8-2 are sample notices of introduction, and Exhibits 8-3 and 8-4 illustrate types of business cards.

Retain the list from the first mailing, and remail periodically. Adding or deleting names and addresses may be necessary occasionally.

The logo shown on the business card can be used on the notice of introduction, also. What logo should you use? A caduceus is appropriate; however, you may wish to be creative and design your own. The use of a logo is not mandatory.

Randolph sent out over 50 letters; the response was minimal. Personal contacts and interviews proved not much better. After a second mailing of letters, people were more willing to become involved with the private practice.[3]

An Accessible Location

A practice may be best located in your home for three reasons. First, it is inexpensive to maintain. Second, it is easily accessible to you. Third, if you live in an average community, it will be accessible to clients.

If you establish practice in a location other than your home, choose a location that is accessible to clients. Locating near a hospital, clinic, health agency, or physician can be beneficial. Be certain there is ample parking and that the practice is visible from the street or that its location is well marked. Clients may be reluctant to visit a practice that is difficult to find or that has no bus service.

Alford and Jensen spent two months looking for office space before opening their private practice. They found it a challenge to locate proper office space. Finally, they found one in a central location and in an area with many elderly people. Geriatrics is their specialty, and the location had adequate parking, busing, and ramps for the handicapped.[4]

Exhibit 8-1 Notice of Introduction

Name of Private Practice
Address
Phone Number(s)

Nursing care and procedures in home or office by professional nurses. Nursing service available by appointment; please telephone at any hour. Referral and consultation with physician when appropriate.

Examples of Nursing Services Available
Catheter care
Colostomy care
Diabetic care
Irrigations
Blood pressure readings
Dressings
Injections
Diet teaching
Stress management
Nutritional counseling

Nursing care is designed to teach the family or client to be independent when possible. Home visits and office visits are available.

Signature
Your Name

Peer Interest and Endorsement

A public service announcement in a local newspaper may help find business partners. It can also be used to publicize your practice or to find nurses with whom you can consult. The support of local peers is comforting. Peer group endorsement, on a larger scale, is supportive, and comforting, and helps the nursing practice flourish.

Many articles have been published regarding private nursing practice in trade journals and general interest magazines. Nurses and the public are not totally unaware of the availability of private practice nursing. However, they need education as to what it is and specifically what your practice provides.

Speaking Engagements

To further inform your community of your practice and its services, you may want to make some oral presentations. Some ideal organizations for

Exhibit 8-2 Notice of Introduction

Name of Private Practice
Address
Phone Number(s)

Hours (List your hours)

This practice is intended to facilitate health care to the public. Professional nursing care is provided in the office, or in clients' homes by professional nurses.

Professional nursing care is provided:

- In collaboration with client's physician where appropriate
- To assist the client's physician
- With the results returned to the client's physician where appropriate
- To teach the client self-care

Examples of Nursing Services

Blood samples	Intravenous
Dressings	Catheter care
Vital signs	Irrigations
Colostomy care	Diabetic care
Injections	Teaching

Please phone the office when the nurse(s) here can be of assistance to you.

Signature
Nurse's Name

Exhibit 8-3 Business Card

Phone Number(s)   Logo

   Practice Name

   Nursing services in home or office. Injections, dressings, catheter, blood pressures, colostomy care, many others.

Hours   Address

Name of Nurse

---

presentations include the Senior Citizen Clubs, Lions Club, Rotary, Parent-Teachers Associations, Masons, Knights of Columbus, Chamber of Commerce, League of Women Voters, Urban League, National Association for the Advancement of Colored People, and others. Speeches to local nursing schools in local colleges can be beneficial.

Exhibit 8-4 Business Card

> Caduceus (Logo)
> 　　　　Your Name or Name of Practice
> Phone Number(s)　　　　　　　　　　　　　　　Address
> Hours

Members of nursing associations may be interested in a presentation during one of their meetings. Nursing associations such as the American Nurses Association, National League for Nursing, Emergency Department Nurses Association, state nursing associations, and local nursing associations may provide the meeting ground. I have discussed the concept of private practice at many of these.

Trade Journals

Preparing an article about your practice and sending it to editors of trade journals will inform peers of your practice. General interest magazines may wish to publish a story regarding your practice; such a story could be of great public interest. They may publish your paper or write about you themselves.

Television

Advertising your practice on television is not called for. However, you may wish to become involved with a news station as it may prepare a health care story regarding your practice. This story would inform local residents that your services exist to aid the public, or that nurses generally provide care to the public.

I appeared on "To Tell the Truth" in 1973. The theme of the show was, "Who is the Private Nurse Practitioner?" This type of media exposure can inform colleagues and the public of what nursing is making available and what your practice has to offer.

Yellow Pages

Undoubtedly, your practice will have at least one telephone. Two may be needed after your clientele increases. Advertisements in the yellow pages of the telephone directory are excellent mechanisms for making your practice known to a great many local residents. Different sizes of advertisements are available, and the telephone representative should be able to aid you in setting up and designing this advertisement.

Public Service Announcements

Placing hard-sell advertisements on radio stations may be illegal and unethical. However, asking several local radio stations to run free, short public service announcements is allowable.

Public service announcements are what they say they are—announcements to the public about a public service. Generally the service is free to the listening public. You could offer free blood pressure readings or another service to senior citizens or other group at your practice during a designated time period.

Radio stations are required by law to periodically run public service announcements on the air. They are short and free; in effect, they inform the public about your practice.

Interviews

Local newspapers or radio stations may wish to interview you so that they can inform their consumers of your story. Interviews are not advertisements, but they can be skillfully employed to send your message to community members.

When Goodspeed began private practice, one objective was to present the concept to the public. The problem was to find an ethical and professional way to advertise. Two interviews published in local newspapers and speeches at several professional gatherings were the answer.[5]

Ripple Effect

As people read or hear about a business, organization, firm, or service, they have a tendency to repeat this news to others who are uninformed. This is called the "ripple effect."

Media publicity leads to word-of-mouth publicity. Word of mouth may be your most valuable form of publicity. Do not neglect to engage in spontaneous conversation or to seize every opportunity to publicize your practice. The ripple effect can be far reaching and long lasting when your message is delivered with sincerity and concern. People will feel compelled to spread the word about your practice, and the effect will continue to gain momentum as time passes.

SUMMARY

Skillful use of available media can greatly improve your publicity, as well as professional and public relations. Be assertive and seek out various routes to promote your practice. If you are meek and reluctant to explore all possible sources of publicity you will probably only hinder the community's awareness of your practice as one of its health care resources.

Alford and Jensen employed announcements in newspapers that were followed up by feature stories. They appeared as guests on talk shows and before various organizations. They had stationery and brochures printed. From all of this effort, they received their reward: referrals and satisfied clients who referred friends and relatives.[6]

McShane and Smith publicized their practice by pounding the pavement. They visited pastors, local schools, police departments, and local organizations to explain their practice. They personally handed out brochures and business cards and also mailed them. This activity not only informed the community about the practice but also informed them about community problems and needs.

The dean of the nursing college they attended sent their brochures to the college's clinical agencies and to other colleges of nursing. Speaking engagements to professional groups were thereby generated, and peer group endorsement was demonstrated.

A psychologist who taught in a local college was a major source of their first referrals. Many of these referrals were for stress management and counseling. Word of mouth was another large source of referrals. Yellow page advertisements and newspaper stories with pictures delivered their public service message to community members. All of these measures helped their practice to grow and serve the community better.[7]

Private practice advertising is a new and assertive role for nurses. Promoting your private practice may feel odd at first, but once you begin, you will enjoy the satisfying results it can have for your community. Informing others of your practice can be exciting because you are promoting health care and providing that very care in a realistic fashion.

NOTES

1. John V. Petrof, Peter S. Carusone, and John E. McDavid, *Small Business Management: Concepts and Techniques for Improving Decisions* (New York: McGraw-Hill Book Company, 1972), p. 343.

2. Harvey R. Cook, *Selecting Advertising Media: A Guide for Small Business* (Washington, D.C.: Small Business Administration, 1969), p. 2–3.

3. Gretchen T. Randolph, "Experiences in Private Practice," *Journal of Psychiatric Nursing and Mental Health Services* 13 (November-December 1975): 16-7.

4. Dolores Marsh Alford and Janet Moll Jensen, "Reflections on Private Practice," *American Journal of Nursing* 76, no. 12 (December 1976): 1967.

5. Harriett E. Goodspeed, "The Independent Practitioner—Can It Survive?" *Journal of Psychiatric Nursing and Mental Health Services* 14 (August 1976): 33.

6. Dolores Marsh Alford and Janet Moll Jensen, "Reflections on Private Practice," *American Journal of Nursing* 76, no. 12 (December 1976): 1967.

7. Nancy Gerberding McShane and Elizabeth McDowell Smith, "Starting a Private Practice in Mental Health Nursing," *American Journal of Nursing* 78, no. 12 (December 1978): 2069–70.

Chapter 9

Model of a Private Practice

IMPRESSIONS

I established private practice in August of 1971. The practice was situated in rented professional office space at a desirable, downtown location. This practice created a first impression in my state that alleviated fears and difficulties of other nurses who may have wanted to practice in a similar fashion.

In preparing a survey of local community health needs for a baccalaureate degree, I realized that a great deal of nursing care was lacking in the community. I met many people while canvassing the community. They all expressed the opinion that nearby, accessible, copious health care was lacking.

Since physicians' offices were overcrowded, and the physicians didn't make house calls, I envisioned that nurses in private practice could make house calls or see clients in their practices. Greater numbers of community members could be seen by health providers, and the health of community members could be upgraded. Nurses practicing from private practice could stress their role as health teachers who provide care similar to that given by physicians early in a health care regimen; later they could overlap roles with physicians. Nurses and physicians could thus collaborate as colleagues, share information, and participate with one another for the clients' benefit.

Role Analysis

Procedure manuals, job analyses, and job descriptions serve to explain the roles nurses perform, and some provide examples of the health care services nurses offer. Nurses can provide these services and many more to clients from a private practice. Traditional roles defining how nurses function and receive remuneration for their services are difficult to modify for roles demanded in contemporary times.

Providers of clients' health needs, practicing from private practice, are able to produce their own job or role analysis. A procedure manual is not necessarily needed. Utilization of quality texts may suffice for procedures. However, your unique roles need your individual attention for creating your role analysis.

Charts and Figures

Organizations can use a chart to visually explain where they fit into the scheme of services in their community. Charts depicting employees' roles in organizations are called organizational charts; they inform employees of their relationship to the organization as a whole and to its other members. Such charts can provide a sense of belonging and a sense of accomplishment.

Create your chart as you see it; it need not be too involved. Figure 9-1 depicts the private practice and the community; the client is the center of the health care. Health care providers and concerned persons encompass the clients; they give them care and support. Figure 9-2, an organizational chart of private practice, shows the nurse/proprietor supervising the practice's staff and caring for the client. Lines indicate flow of communication in each chart.

Nursing Process

The example of nursing processes you utilize will depend on your educational or literature sources, empirical knowledge, understanding of your clients' needs, and image of nursing. The process of nursing is the key to individualized care. As you gain experience in private practice, you will acquire a progression of skills that enable you to provide more sophisticated care. Developing and employing a nursing process is necessary to ensure safe and proficient care to your clients.

Generally, processes of nursing contain these phases, in this sequence: assess, plan, implement, evaluate, and audit. The application is inherent in your professional role. If you have difficulty with the nursing process, refrain from private practice until you are capable of employing it safely. Figure 9-3 illustrates a nursing process.

According to Murchison, Nicholas, and Hanson, the nursing process was created in response to the need to apply nursing practice logically and orderly. It provides a structure through which nurses can provide optimum care. No set of rules applies for all situations. Decisions are derived from the interdisciplinary approach that is characteristic of professional conduct.[1]

Figure 9-1 Chart Depicting the Client and Private Practice in the Community

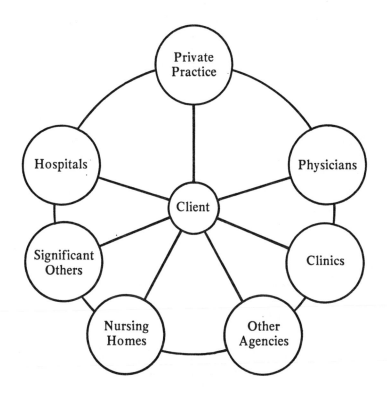

Lines show possible channels of communication

Nursing Versus Medical Role

Nurses' and physicians' roles constantly overlap. This interfacing of roles varies in degree, depending upon the clients' needs, the nurses' capabilities, and the care provided. Propinquity of the roles of nurses and physicians should not threaten either, since the roles have always overlapped to some degree. Lately, this overlap has increased, and in private practice it will increase even more.

Nurses entering private practice are not expected to expand their roles out of nursing and into medicine, but are expected to maintain, develop, and practice their current roles to their fullest extent. At times private nurse

Figure 9-2 Organizational Chart of Private Practice

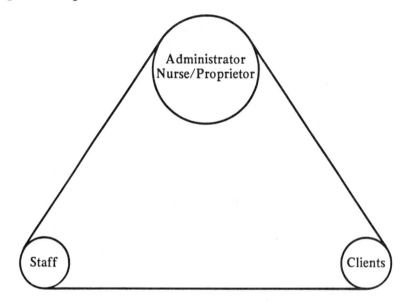

Lines show possible channels of communication

Note: Staff may be further subdivided if it includes many individuals with
varied health care delivery skills, experience, education, and responsibilities.

---

practitioners will be expected to expand their roles so that they interface with
physicians' roles to a greater extent.

According to Lynaugh and Bates, nurses and physicians are two subcul-
tures, and the gap between them is seen in different ways. Often nurses and
physicians use different terms for the same thing. This practice can create a
gap in communication, which can be bridged by translating the words each
uses. One process may be perceived differently by nurses and doctors. Transla-
tions are not useful here, and nurses and physicians thus confuse, alienate, and
antagonize one another.[2]

Two terms that nurses and physicians accept from each other without too
much difficulty are *home visit,* a term customarily reserved for nurses, and
house call, a term ordinarily reserved for physicians.

Figure 9-3 The Nursing Process

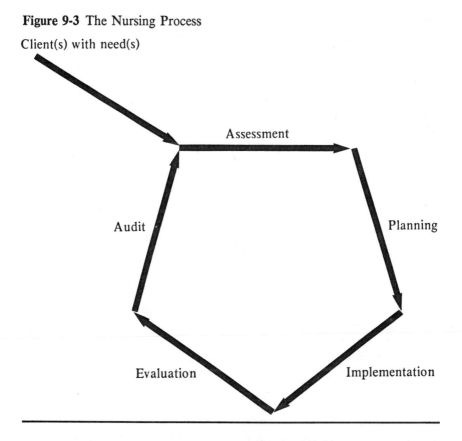

Two terms used to demonstrate differences between the two professions are *problem* or *need* versus *diagnosis.* The nurse would say that the client's problem or need is such and such, and the physician would say the client's diagnosis is such and such. These words have specific professional territory; at times they lead to contention between the professions. Nurses and physicians must become flexible regarding territorial rights, since the members of each of these professions may be working together more closely and appropriately performing some roles that customarily may have been in the other's territory. These roles relate to terminology and services. Since health care is more sophisticated because of modern technological advances, the members of each profession, nursing and medicine, must employ one another's expertise for clients' health care regimens. It is possible that an identical function could be considered the practice of nursing when provided by a nurse and the practice of medicine when provided by a physician. Figure 9-4 illustrates how roles overlap. Table 9-1 compares a nursing model with a medical model.

Figure 9-4 Interface of Nurses' and Physicians' Roles

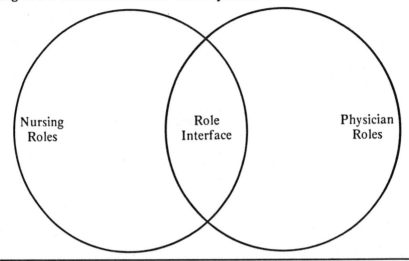

No contention by either profession should exist when nursing and medical roles are applied judiciously. The majority of the elements shown in either model relate primarily to private practice; however, they can be modified and transferred to other health care settings. Thus, elements not shown in either model, but existent in other health care settings, can be modified and transferred into private practice.

Individual private nurse practitioners will need to customize this nursing model to apply to their private practice, community needs, skills, and capabilities. Only moderate customizing is advised to ensure quality control. Figure 9-5 illustrates a model of a private nursing practice.

According to Henderson, the process of arriving at a diagnosis is the same for nurses as it is for physicians. The terminology in the diagnosis is what distinguishes nursing from medicine. Each profession is interested in assessing clients and identifying their needs.

Physicians are concerned with diagnosis and treatment of a disease. This treatment is directed at the cause or symptoms of that disease. Nursing is concerned with diagnosis and treatment of human response to environmental stressors; treatment is directed to the etiology of the response.[3]

In arriving at diagnoses and preparing regimens of care, each profession undergoes similar processes. In actual implementation or provision of care, each profession has a territory of services reserved for itself. This territory can be entered by the other professional when the professional is competent to do so, the client's regimen calls for it, and it is legally permissible.

Figure 9-5 Model of a Private Nursing Practice

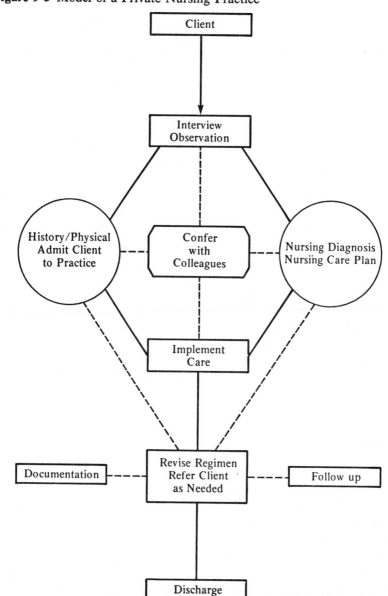

Solid lines indicate direct channels of communication.
Broken lines indicate indirect channels of communication.

Table 9-1 Comparison of the Nursing Model and the Medical Model

Nursing Model	Medical Model
1. Interview and observe client.	1. Assess client.
2. Refer client to another health care provider if necessary.	2. Refer client to another health care provider if necessary.
3. Admit community member as a client in the private practice.	3. Admit community member as a client in the private practice.
4. Obtain history, recognize needs, and make physical exam.	4. Obtain history, determine needs, and make physical exam.
5. Refer client if indicated.	5. Refer client if indicated.
6. Make a nursing diagnosis.	6. Make a medical diagnosis.
7. Confer with client's physician.	7. Confer with client's nurse.
8. Develop a plan of nursing care. Write orders.	8. Develop a plan of medical care. Write orders.
9. Implement nursing care plan; collaborate with client's physician as needed.	9. Implement medical care plan; collaborate with client's nurse as needed.
10. Confer with colleagues, observe client progress. Refer client to another health care provider if necessary.	10. Confer with colleagues, observe client progress. Refer client to another health care provider if necessary.
11. Confer with client's physician when appropriate.	11. Confer with client's nurse when appropriate.
12. Revise nursing care plan or nursing regimen as needed.	12. Revise medical care plan as needed.
13. Refer client if necessary.	13. Refer client if necessary.
14. Document client's care and progress in nursing notes, throughout all stages of contact with client.	14. Document client's care and progress in medical notes, throughout all stages of contact with client.
15. Plan for discharge of client.	15. Plan for discharge of client.
16. Discharge; write discharge summary.	16. Discharge; write discharge summary.
17. Give follow-up care if indicated.	17. Give follow-up care if indicated.

SUMMARY

Nursing and medicine can work together to enhance clients' care. The cooperation they could realize may not be so difficult to achieve.

The nursing model is very similar to the medical model. Both professions need to understand and accept this reality. As nurses enter private practice in larger numbers, the gap between services provided by nurses and physicians will be reduced.

If you enter private practice, develop your own model of practice. Each organization or private practice has its own unique personality and character. This model reflects you and how you envision your practice.

NOTES

1. Irene Murchison, Thomas S. Nicholas, and Rachel Hanson, *Legal Accountability in the Nursing Process* (Saint Louis: The C. V. Mosby Company, 1978), p. 2–3.

2. Joan E. Lynaugh and Barbara Bates, "The Two Languages of Nursing and Medicine," *American Journal of Nursing* 73, no. 1 (January 1973): 66.

3. Betty Henderson, R.N., M.N., "Nursing Diagnosis: Theory and Practice," *Advances in Nursing Science,* 1, no. 1 (October 1978): 82–3.

Part III

Practice Management for Nurse Practitioners

Chapter 10

Private Practice as a Business

SELF-PROPRIETORSHIP

A private nurse practitioner or self-employed nurse has many advantages not available in traditional employment settings. Perhaps the greatest advantage is the close contact it affords with clients, colleagues, the public, employees, and suppliers. Nurses in private practice perform an individualized service since they have an intimate knowledge of the community and client.

Ganong and Ganong say that in private practice you, the nurse, are the center of your work world. You and your employment situation are special. Your work world is more you than anything else. You have greater influence, responsibility, authority, and control in your work world than you realize or use. Nurses frequently lose sight of this. The individual nurse has the responsibility for initiating decision-making authority. The organizational relationships in traditional employment settings make initiating authority difficult for nurses; this difficulty often leads to role ambiguity.[1]

Developing and managing your private practice will enhance your authority and responsibility to a level that enables you to practice nursing with less role ambiguity. Your decision-making ability will be strengthened as will your authority and ability to deliver increased and more positive nursing care. You will be taking the initiative to deliver quality and needed nursing care.

According to Tate and colleagues, self-proprietorship comprises a source of new processes, ideas, and services that large institutions are reluctant to provide. Large enterprises are not as flexible as small ones. Small enterprises encourage competition not only in price but also in design, efficiency, and quality of service. Independent business is a basic American freedom. People entering it have greater freedom to make decisions and to provide a wider variety of services. This freedom yields zest and genuine interest in one's work, and it teaches people to become more efficient leaders. Small businesses enable the workers to employ their special abilities in a more effective way.[2]

Along with the advantages of self-proprietorship come problems. Many nurses may not possess enough experience and money to enter the business world. Some other potential problems are: selecting a poor location, poor planning, mismanaging finances, purchasing too many capital goods, possessing the wrong attitudes, withholding too much revenue for yourself, and letting the misconceptions of private practice cloud intelligent and proper management.

The best way to cope with these potential disadvantages is to recognize your limitations; investigate and plan; keep adequate records; be cognizant of your cash flow; and seek professional guidance from your attorney, accountant, peers, colleagues, banker, and others. Remember that any business venture has its ups and downs. The entire endeavor will be a learning process with trial and error often being the rule of thumb.

Managing and owning your own practice can enable you to fulfill some of your needs. A great deal of this depends upon the type of person you are and the dedication you have to your business. Owning a private nursing practice can reward you by providing:

- reduced role ambiguity
- greater authority
- greater decision-making opportunities
- a passageway for practicing nursing to its fullest extent
- increased income
- satisfying services to clients
- community prestige
- new challenges, experiences, and skills
- an opportunity to take pride in your practice and yourself

Planning

Planning is fundamental but often taken for granted. Planning is a vital, beginning step in administration or management. You may want to design a master plan to guide your business; your goals and philosophies exert much influence on your planning.

Some beginning considerations include:

- studying of the market for your business (community needs)
- determining the geographic boundaries of your service area
- deciding the types of services you will provide
- finding a location
- meeting start-up costs (capital requirements)
- preparing of a budget

- researching other private nursing practices
- setting goals and defining philosophy
- purchasing equipment and materials
- finding partners
- choosing advisors
- setting up

Your plans are guidelines that may change constantly. They can help you in starting out and in continued management of your nursing practice. Your plans can be either long or short range. They are intended to aid in decision making and in progress.

According to Subrin, there are few, if any, answers on how to begin a business. Nurses who wish to enter the business world should research available literature, seek professional advice, plan, and think through the results of various decisions. The personal and professional rewards from establishing a private practice will probably outweigh the additional responsibilities.[3] Planning consists of the following steps:

1. Recognize and state the problem or goal.
2. Compile relevant facts.
3. Establish alternative courses of action.
4. Evaluate the pros and cons to alternative courses of action.
5. Select a plan.
6. Reconnoiter and adjust the plan as needed.

To ensure that your plans are complete, you should be able to answer the following questions:

- Why this plan?
- What action is needed to carry it out?
- Where will this action take place?
- Who will carry it out?
- How shall it be carried out?
- How stringently should it be carried out?

Your time is invaluable; be sure to plan it well so that you can manage your practice effectively. To aid in planning your time, consider:

- Should this activity be eliminated or delegated?
- Should this activity be combined with others?
- Can the time required for this function be reduced?
- Should the sequence of functions be rearranged?

- Can the activities be organized better?
- Have someone (a secretary if you employ one) establish the priority of mail, incoming calls, appointments, and activities. Adhere to appointment schedules.

After all of the planning, contemplating, counseling, thinking, asking, and canvassing, decide on a location and set up for practice. Prepare your practice by installing equipment and materials. Provide treatment rooms, a waiting room, an office, and perhaps a library. Have a telephone, adequate lighting, and bathrooms installed.

In the event you should have to relocate your practice, be certain to inform your clients and your public adequately. Relocating does not have to be deleterious, provided you inform others of your move.

Nurse-Provider

In the past the term provider was not applied to the nurse. However, nurses are primary and major providers of health care to the public and are providers in the same sense that physicians and other health care providers are.

Before delivering client care, the nurse-provider should inform clients or their families about services, office hours, fees, home visits, and office visits. A referring physician, hospital, agency, or person also needs to know this information.

To determine whether you can deliver requested care, obtain as much data as possible: the client's name, address, phone number, diagnosis, needs, and the client's physician's name, address, and phone number. Contact the client or physician for appropriate information. Once needs and materials are determined and obtained, you can provide your professional care.

PRIVATE PRACTICE AS A PROFIT-MAKING BUSINESS

The concept of nurses being self-employed, billing clients directly, and working for profit is new; it can be somewhat uncomfortable to some nurses. Nurses working in hospitals and other institutions receive payment for their services on the basis of the 8-hour shift, as either part- or full-time employees. In these institutions, the client pays the nurses for their services, but indirectly. (The client pays the institution, and the institution pays the nurse.) Although nurses employed in traditional institutions do not work on a fee-for-service basis, the client's health insurance pays the institution for the nursing care on a fee-for-service basis.

Health insurance will not pay nurses from your nursing practice on a fee-for-service basis. Clients must be billed directly from private practice and they must pay their bills to the practice. Many clients are willing to purchase your specialized services regardless of whether their insurance covers the cost. Clients pay nurses for their services on a fee-for-service basis because it provides the care they want, when they want it, and where they want it. Nurses in private practice provide a closer, more personalized touch and can keep clients at home with loved ones.

Generally, nurses have no problem receiving payment; clients are accustomed to receiving and paying bills from their health care providers. Nurses need to gain a similar feeling. Billing for nursing services is a professional role nurses are not yet accustomed to.

The nursing profession should realize that to be a charitable profession will only inhibit nursing's future and ability to extend care to people. Each individual nurse needs to generate enough revenue from the nursing profession to remain alive and healthy enough to practice competent nursing. From this revenue comes the continued education that benefits the public. Transportation and other costs of being a nurse must also be met. Without proper remuneration, nurses cannot nurse properly.

According to Nordberg and King, physicians and hospitals have received third-party payment for a long time. Usually one-half of their income is realized from these payments. Only lately have third-parties begun to reimburse for services provided by other health care providers. Individual nurses will not necessarily receive third-party payment.[4]

According to Rodin, nursing salaries are not as high as they should be for the amount of education required to be a nurse. Salaries are improving. People do not enter nursing to get rich; they generally have more idealistic views of nursing. Many pathways are now available for nurses to put their idealism to work.[5]

If nursing schools were to expose students to the billing system of health care and teach that nurses can bill clients fee-for-service, nurses could accept the direct service payment system so many other health care providers use. In some cases when there is an indigent client, the care can be provided gratis.

In spite of providing gratis care on occasion and not receiving third-party payment, there should be enough clients to get your practice to be a going concern. Nurses and the nursing profession are unquestionably a sine qua non. Nurses are essential to health care, and private nursing practices can enhance health care.

Group or Single Practice?

You can manage your practice by yourself (a single practice) or form a group of owners or partners (group practice). Some advantages of a single practice are sole ownership and therefore no bickering in making decisions. Single practices may be smaller and easier to manage. Clients may prefer them since they tend to receive a greater personal touch in them. In a single practice, you have to meet your clients' and your needs only. On the other hand, single practices afford less aid in decision making. You receive less emotional support. You bear costs and problems alone. In the event you are ill, services go unprovided, although for vacation, holiday, and illness, you can arrange with another nurse to cover your practice. You may have less free time.

The burden of costs, problems, and decisions can be shared in a group practice. When a member of the group gets sick, another group member can easily fill in. Group members can provide emotional support to the others. Decision making is sometimes more difficult, as group members may not be able to agree. In-fighting and professional jealousy might occur, which would be destructive to the practice. Some group members may not carry their share of the work or responsibility. Responsibilities and authority should be clarified in the early stages of the practice.

Nurse/Administrator

The nurse in private practice must become a manager almost overnight. Getting into the business of private practice is a good way to learn business management. Although practical experience is often the best teacher, management courses regarding private practice could prove helpful. Most nurses could benefit from a course in personnel management, as nurses at all levels must advise and direct aides, orderlies, technicians, and others regarding client care and protocol.

The terms manager and administrator are almost synonymous. Mistakes help you to learn and improve your management skills. Administrative skills are learned through trial and error.

According to Hopper, nursing administrators are essential to all areas of nursing. A nurse can become an administrator by learning about administration in formal education and by landing a job as an administrator. Some practices of being an administrator cannot be learned in classrooms. Many people become administrators without formal education; their education is derived from actual experience. You have to develop your management style.[6]

According to Mooth and Ritva, supervision should not stem only from the person carrying the title of supervisor. The responsibility for it is inherent in all of the nursing positions from the director of nurses to the staff nurse, whether those entitled supervisor realize it or not.[7]

Nurses who take this responsibility develop their administrative skills greatly. Donovan says that nurses have been administrators for a long time, although this has often gone unrecognized. Nurses and administrators need to scrutinize this issue more thoughtfully.[8]

Kron contends that leadership is needed in all nursing services. Nurses perform administrative roles whether they are staff nurses or directors of nursing. Leadership helps to create changes in people.[9] A change to more dynamic leadership would give nursing the opportunity to improve.

Layout

The physical size of a new practice should be moderate. Going overboard in size may push costs up too high and be difficult to manage, especially at first. It should be large enough to enable you to work in it, though, and a little extra room at first may be wise because it will allow for growth of your practice.

The location of various areas can be important; a treatment room should not be next to the front door. The waiting room belongs near the front door. The next area could be your reception area, which could be combined with the office. Treatment rooms could follow with bathrooms nearby. The library could also be nearby. Juxtapose the design to find an arrangement that works for your floor plan.

Hours

The hours that your practice is open are determined by you and your coworkers. You can be open as many or as few hours per week as you wish. Physicians' practices are open through the week at staggered hours. They also work by appointment. This concept can apply well to nursing practices. The staggered hour system works especially well if you have a traditional nursing job while managing your practice. There would be no conflict of interests, if staggered hours existed.

Staggering hours means opening different hours each day; for example, Monday, Wednesday, and Friday—5:00 P.M. to 9:00 P.M.; Tuesday and Saturday—10:00 A.M. to 8:00 P.M. If you need to change hours, the key is to inform your clients of the change. Be certain to post your hours, phone number(s), and business name where the public can see them easily.

Saturday and evening hours facilitate visits from clients who could not come during standard work hours. Remember that you can schedule your home visits around traditional employment and staggered office hours. This, too, enables you to reach more people.

Schedule your appointments according to the amount of time each will take. When your practice is closed, you can receive incoming phone calls by telephone answering machine or by hiring an answering service. Both are effective.

Exhibit 10-1 History Form

Name of Nursing Practice
Street
Town

Phone(s)   Hours

Date_____

Client's Name: _____ Phone No.: _____
Client's Address: _____
Ht. _____ Wt. _____ Age _____ Sex _____
D.O.B. _____ Marital Status _____
Referred by: _____ Client's Physician _____
Present Illness:

Family History:

Personal History:

Current Medications:

Current Physician's Orders:

Vital Signs:

                                                    Nurse: _____·___

When calls come in regarding emergency care and you are closed, the caller could telephone the police, an emergency department, or ambulance.

Forms

Having forms preprinted is easy, inexpensive, and adds a professional air to your practice. Such forms would include a history form and a nursing note form. Exhibit 10-1 shows a sample history form, and Exhibit 10-2, a sample nurse's note. These forms offer uniformity of client data and are easy to work with. They enable you to keep neat, organized, and easily obtainable records.

Exhibit 10-2 Nurse's Notes

Name of Nursing Practice
Address

Client's Physician _____

Client's Name: _____ Address _____

Client's Telephone Number: _____

Date and Time _____ Record of Nursing Care:

_____

Equipment

Stock a new practice with the equipment you feel you will use most frequently. Much of this equipment will be for the office, not just for client care. Some equipment you should consider obtaining is listed below.

Waiting Room

- two or three benches
- chairs
- garbage cans
- ash trays
- magazines and a magazine stand
- flowers in pots
- music system
- coat rack
- pictures

Office/Reception Room

- desk and chair
- chairs for clients
- telephone
- file cabinets
- garbage can
- coat rack
- pictures
- ash trays
- telephone answering machine
- fire extinguisher

Treatment Rooms and Waiting Area

- shelving to store supplies
- examining table
- scale
- vital signs equipment
- gowns
- cleaning material for used equipment
- sink
- door to the treatment room to ensure privacy
- adequate lighting
- gooseneck lamps

Library

The library is for staff use, to aid in the delivery of care.

- shelving
- tables
- chairs
- lighting
- books and magazines related to health care

Bathroom

- toilet material
- cleaning equipment
- mirror
- shelf

Nursing Equipment

This will vary from specialty to specialty, but much of the following will be needed:

- thermometer
- sphygmomanometer
- sterile bandages
- dressing material
- tape
- gauze
- dressing packs
- sterile Q-tips
- catheter tray
- irrigating set

- emergency kit
- resuscitator

Keeping medications and syringes in the office is not needed. Clients can bring these with them when they visit the practice. Medications and syringes would be in the client's home already, when you made a home visit.

When you do keep medications and syringes in your practice, have a safe place to lock them up. A file cabinet, desk, or safe will secure them. A metal enclosure is better than plastic or wood. Lock refrigerated medications in refrigerators. Use quality locks, and install burglar alarms if needed.

If the majority of your care is by appointment, you will not have to keep too much more equipment on hand. Determining client needs ahead of time, when making the appointment, enables you to purchase the exact equipment before the appointment.

When setting up their practice, McShane and Smith bought office equipment from second-hand stores; they painted much of it themselves. They also borrowed equipment. This equipment ranged from various types of chairs to lamps, draperies, and a large coffee pot. They have a large waiting room, two small offices, and a bathroom. Their practice is on the entire first floor of an office building on a main street. The rent is reasonable, and they are near a bus stop, parking, and the train station.[10]

Uniforms

Your code of dress is entirely up to you. You can wear your nursing uniform or street clothes. You do not have to purchase a new wardrobe of uniforms. Wearing street clothes in good taste should be accepted by clients. Your behavior will identify you to others as a nurse. However, it is best to always identify yourself to others and clients as the nurse. A name badge can be effective.

Policy Manual

Whether your practice demands a policy manual will become apparent once it is underway. In some cases, a policy manual may be needed before business gets underway. Early planning can help you to prepare one. At any rate, a working model should be in your head, as a tool. A policy manual is most needed for a very large office with many employees or a practice with a great turnover of personnel.

Taxes

Finances require careful control, or they will soon get out of hand. Save receipts from all of your expenses. At each year's end you will be able to claim several of your expenses for tax deductions. Annual taxes should be completed by an accountant who is familiar with the claims you can make and with the long tax form. If possible, keep the same accountant year after year as this will enable your accountant to become familiar with your practice and thus advise and guide you better. Plus, each year your claims and forms may become more involved.

A log of all business-related phone calls and business-related miles traveled is useful. Having a second and separate telephone for the business is a good way to itemize calls. Your expenses are claimed against your taxable income, thus reducing your taxable income. This is the government's way of helping all businesses recapture some of their spent money.

Office equipment may be depreciated in value, and amortizing may be needed. This expertise, too, is a special skill offered by an accountant. Each year you can deduct the prior year's accountant's fees, thereby adding to your claims.

Going Concern

Once you wend your way through the start-up costs and problems, you can begin to relax and enjoy the daily business of managing your practice and delivering nursing care. Start-up work does not take forever; usually only a few months are required. It comes with all businesses at the beginning.

Your rewards will begin in caring for your first client; they come in the form of an inner sense of accomplishment. To know that you are really helping a person in your unique way is a great satisfaction. Experiencing this feeling of reward should make all of the initial work worth it.

Running any business is work, but many people do it for the sense of freedom and accomplishment it affords. Private practice is a new, healthy, and exciting role for nurses. Your enthusiasm will rub off onto others, and many of them will want to help you even in the smallest of ways.

After that first client, others will follow. As more and more clients visit you, your practice will become self-supporting. Once your practice is a going concern, you may wish to consider moving to a larger location, or expanding to a second location. The second location could be in a nearby town or community.

SUMMARY

Nurses should recognize the expansion of community hospitals as an indicator of the need for additional health care in that community. Hospitals as service providers are a big business.

Now is the time for a change in nursing from the meek and passive to a more affirmative role. This affirmative role can be achieved by incorporating a business climate into the nursing profession.

As nurses and nursing accept the concept of private practice, a greater recognition and utilization of nurses will be realized. This greater recognition and utilization can only benefit the public.

Self-proprietorship nursing yields many benefits for the public. Perhaps the greatest is that clients and families can have a family nurse, one of their choice. This choice has been kept from the public for far too long.

Nursing has long been a big business; however, the nurses and the public have not had direct control of it. Others have contained nursing to a suppressed level of service. This suppression has met the needs of others and made large profits for them. As nurses become more assertive and business-oriented, these needs and rewards will go to whom they rightfully belong—the clients and the nurses.

NOTES

1. Joan M. Ganong, R.N., M.S. and Warren L. Ganong, C.M.C., *Nursing Management* (Germantown, Maryland: Aspen Systems Corporation, 1976), pp. 6–7.

2. Curtis E. Tate, Jr. et al., *The Complete Guide to Your Own Business* (Homewood, Illinois: Dow Jones-Irwin, 1977), p. 5.

3. Lawrence I. Subrin, C.P.A., "The Business Aspects of Private Practice," *Journal of Nursing Administration* 7, no. 7 (September 1977): 51.

4. Beatrice Nordberg and Lynelle King, "Third-Party Payment for Patient Education," *American Journal of Nursing* 76, no. 8 (August 1976): 1276.

5. Rita Rodin, "Today's Florence Nightingales, Everything's Changed But the Idealism," *Working Woman* 3 (May 1978): 35.

6. Susan Hopper, "Becoming an Administrator Overnight!" *Nursing Outlook* 23, no. 12 (December 1975): 752.

7. A. Mooth and M. Ritva, *Developing the Supervisory Skills of the Nurse: A Behavioral Science Approach* (New York: Macmillan, 1966), pp. 13–14.

8. Helen M. Donovan, *Nursing Service Administration Managing the Enterprise* (Saint Louis: The C. V. Mosby Company, 1975), p. 3.

9. Thora Kron, R.N., B.S., "How to Become a Better Leader," *Nursing 76* 6, no. 10 (October 1976): 67.

10. Nancy Gerberding McShane, and Elizabeth McDowell Smith, "Starting a Private Practice in Mental Health Nursing," *American Journal of Nursing* 78, no. 12 (December 1978): 2068–9.

Chapter 11

Financial Management

PECUNIARY AFFAIRS

The costs of setting up a practice can become out-of-hand. To prevent or minimize this, provide time for thinking, planning, and taking action regarding your finances. Economic environment plays a vital role in your success, so peruse it carefully. Be certain to estimate the amount of capital you will need, how long it will take to recoup your start-up costs or investment, and how long it will take to reach an acceptable level of income. Though answers to the questions will not necessarily be accurate, giving them consideration and planning can keep you from serious financial difficulty.

You may also have to determine how you will live until your practice becomes a going concern. It may be wise to maintain traditional nursing employment during start-up time. Traditional employment could be maintained as long as desired, provided it did not conflict with your practice. Many business people manage their own business and are employed elsewhere.

Utilize your own resources and those of others who are in similar business ventures. These people can include private nurse practitioners, physicians, dentists, physical therapists, chiropractors, and other health care providers in private practice. Your banker, lawyer, accountant, or bookkeeper may also be able to advise you.

Start-up Fees

All businesses incur beginning costs. Eventually they will be returned to you, provided your practice is successful. A portion of these start-up fees may be incorporated into your fees for your service. This practice enables you to obtain gainful returns in relation to your initial investments. Businesses do this, as it is sound business practice.

Some start-up costs may take a few years to recoup. The length of time depends on the depreciation schedule you employ for purchased equipment, the activity of your practice, and inflation. Once your practice gets going and you have recovered many of your start-up costs, you may not want to lower your fees for services as your maintenance costs may be reflected in them. In fact, fees may have to be raised many times because of inflation.

Agree reports that start-up costs and operating costs vary with the different services offered by private nurse practitioners. These initial investments can range from $150 to $15,000. Operating costs can vary from $45 a month to $550 a month.[1]

Budgets

Start-up fees and maintenance fees can be planned for through the use of budgeting. Preparing a well-thought-out budget should receive top priority. A stringent budget will facilitate control of finances and give the practice an even greater chance for success.

Budgets are as reliable as those who compile them. You need not be an accounting major to prepare a budget for your practice. Often you have more personal resources than you realize.

Preparing short-range and long-range budgets may prove useful. Budgets need to be adjusted on occasion; however, the more stringent they are, the better. Avoid becoming so stringent that you do not spend revenue for necessities. Be prepared to purchase when the time is ripe, even when the cost may be a little more than you budgeted. Your purchase may prove a worthy investment overall.

For example, if you want a location in an area that has nearby health care providers, say in a professional building near a clinic or hospital, but no space is available, you may budget your funds for a less desirable space. Before you take the less desirable location, the first choice may become available, but at a higher rent than you budgeted for. It may be to your advantage to readjust your budget so that you can set up your practice at the more attractive location.

The budget should have funds in a section called unexpected costs or miscellaneous funds. Appropriation of such funds could enable you to purchase the right thing at the right time. Renting the cheaper dwelling could save you a sizable disbursement of costs per year in rent. Renting the more desirable, but more expensive, dwelling may produce an additional source of revenue because its location increases public and colleague awareness, availability, and use. The additional revenue produced from the more expensive location may be enough to enable you to come out financially ahead. Also, the more desirable location could afford faster growth of your practice.

To obtain maximum results, the budget process should be continuous. Efficient operation of your practice can be achieved only by adopting a business viewpoint with regard to expenditures and management. Budgetary control is required.

Choosing from among your many needs will be one of your major responsibilities. The decision on what items to include in a budget involves determining the relative values of the competing needs. A decision to include one item may mean the exclusion of another. There is no absolute right or wrong as a value standard. The results of appropriating funds in a budget for one item must be more valuable than the results if funds were used for another item. You will not be expected to meet all of the demands you may encounter. Some will need to be deleted; you must make a decision.

Compute and compile your needs, gather budget data, establish your budget, review it periodically, and adjust it accordingly. Use your budget as a planning device, a tool for financial management. It also serves as a means of evaluating the direction of your private practice.

Table 11-1 demonstrates a suggested budget outline. You must provide the financial values and establish the time period.

Books

A new set of books should be opened for the business, whether it is professionally corporated or not. The aid of an accountant or bookkeeper should be sought. These professionals help you set up the accounts in your new books.

Establish a new banking and checking account for the business. Remember, although you own the business, it is a separate entity, corporated or not, from you. You can draw a salary as an employee of that business.

Financial Assistance

Subrin explains that you should try to appropriate sufficient funds to pay for the start-up costs and expenses for up to six months. Loans are a normal proceeding in the business world. Borrowing funds is common practice for amassing funds in advance of need. Your budgets and books will aid you in demonstrating need and security to loan officers.[2]

Sources of funds can be personal: from individuals, private investment companies, various types of banks, government lending programs, small business investment companies, business development companies, loan companies, and equipment finance companies. Whatever you utilize, it is wise to investigate all sources regarding interest charges, loan periods, and other regulations.

The amount of money borrowed should allow for the unexpected. Payment terms should be amounts your budget calculates you will be able to meet.

Table 11-1 Private Practice Budget Outline

Rent
1. Security deposit
Utilities
1. Electric
2. Telephone
3. Gas, oil, heat
Salaries and taxes
1. Yours
2. Employees'
3. Business taxes
4. FICA
5. Workmen's compensation
Equipment
1. Furnishings
2. Maintenance
3. Supplies
Advertising
1. The shingle
2. Business cards
3. Notice of introduction
Stationery
1. Forms
2. Postage
Building renovation and maintenance
Insurance
1. Malpractice
2. General
Professional corporation costs
Moving costs
Automobile use
1. Mileage
2. Gas
3. Wear and tear
4. Insurance
5. Maintenance
Education
1. Formal
2. Self-study
Consultation
1. Formal

2. Informal
Miscellaneous

Analyze these costs in relation to the following sources of funds to realize capital investment needs as they relate to private nursing practice.
Funds available from:
1. Personal savings
2. Borrowed
3. Traditional employment
4. Received from services rendered through private practice
   a. Nursing care
   b. Consultation to potential private nurse practitioners

You may be able to obtain free assistance from the Small Business Administration (SBA), a government program for small businesses. Contact the SBA at the nearest field office. It may make low-interest loans to your practice. Consulting with others, utilizing loans, doing some research, and preparing should enable you to manage your finances well.

Rented Versus In-Home Locations

Rent and security deposits comprise a significant portion of your start-up fees. Rent alone comprises a large ongoing expense, perhaps the largest. If you are a home owner and have a mortgage to meet, the additional rent for your practice may be prohibitive. If you rent a home or an apartment, additional rent charges for a practice may be too constraining. To reduce the overhead incurred if you were to support two dwellings, you could locate your practice in your home. To locate it in your apartment may not be possible because of space considerations, but a home may have enough extra room to set up a private practice.

It would be less constraining financially to set your practice up in your home. The concept of professional persons practicing from their homes is legal and widely accepted. Physicians, dentists, lawyers, insurance agents, and other professional people commonly practice from a home setting. Home practices are convenient; you have no problem in getting there.

Business zoning laws may prohibit an in-home practice. Research this beforehand, because you may be able to purchase a permit to practice your profession in your residential zone.

Some negative aspects to an in-home practice are that you may lose some needed space in your home. Your privacy at home may be slightly interrupted, and the renovations, if any, may hinder you. Also, locating on another site may draw more clients than an in-home practice.

The advantages of an in-home practice often outweigh the disadvantages. The primary advantages of an in-home practice, again, are the savings in rent payments and your accessibility to your practice. The need for renovation may be low.

Two points you need to weigh carefully are the in-home rent savings and the out-of-home public awareness. Whichever you choose, be certain to give each careful consideration, as they both reflect ultimate finances, which may make or break your practice.

Equipment, Supplies, and Furnishings

Costs for equipment, supplies, and furnishings can run high, especially in the beginning. Once you have purchased your equipment and supplies, maintaining them is less expensive. If you shop frugally, purchase used material, receive donations, or use things already on hand, you will be able to keep these costs to a minimum.

Equipment, for example, consists of stethescopes, sphygmomanometers, scales, basins, thermometers, various lights, treatment tables, waste containers, and stools. Supplies, for example, consist of syringes, alcohol sponges, sterile dressing material, colostomy material, blood tubes, tourniquets, needles, catheter care material, chux, sterile gloves, and stationery. Furnishings, for example, consist of chairs, desks, file cabinets, shelving, telephone answering machine or service, telephone, coat racks, benches, ash trays, curtains, the shingle, music, lighting, magazines, book shelves, locked cabinets, and wastebaskets.

The materials cited are commonly needed. Purchase enough to get your practice going; do not overpurchase. Purchasing in small amounts at first is wise. Since care is often by appointment, you have time to gather needed material. Thus, you can avoid overpurchasing.

Renovation

Setting up a practice area may require slight structural changes. You may have to add a sink or a bathroom or panel off a treatment room, reception area, or waiting room. Shop around for materials that are low cost or on sale. Hire plumbers, carpenters, or electricians who charge reasonable rates. A friend, neighbor, or relative may be able to renovate for you without charge.

Insurance

At least two types of insurance should be considered: malpractice and general. General insurance covers fire, theft, and accidents. Consulting with a reputable insurance broker regarding insurance is wise.

Insurance is usually not a prerequisite to practicing your profession from your private practice. Be sure to research this, though, for the laws applying to you. A smart nurse would probably secure both types; knowledgeable nurses who do not enter private practice often purchase malpractice insurance anyway.

The costs for either type of insurance are usually minimal and not constraining. Insurance provides financial security to you and your assets. Often, the malpractice insurance that you have before going into private practice applies automatically to your practicing as a nurse from a private practice. Securing malpractice insurance on yourself covers malpractice as a nurse regardless of the institutions, agencies, offices, practices, or locations from which you practice nursing.

Malpractice insurance can be obtained from several sources. A local insurance broker could advise you, the telephone book could inform you, or other nurses could aid you. Various nursing associations could also advise you of how to obtain it. Shopping around and comparing various types of malpractice insurance could prove beneficial.

Printed Matter

Forms for use in your practice's office can be designed and printed. Printed forms have a neat and professional appearance. The cost is low, well worth the consistency, organization, and professionalism they afford. A nearby printer with whom you can develop a business relationship may be the best.

Maintenance Fees

These costs occur constantly. Maintenance fees are usually calculated on a monthly basis. They include utilities, such as heating, air conditioning, water, and electricity; the telephone, wages, repairs, equipment, supplies, or furnishings; postage, stationery, insurance, printing, gasoline, car insurance, wear and tear on the car, and mileage. These fees may be calculated either on an ongoing or on a depreciated basis.

Fees for your services have your start-up and maintenance costs included along with profit. Keep accurate records of your maintenance costs, and incorporate them into your budget.

Generating Revenue

Your fee schedule should contain reasonable charges to clients, but should not be demeaning to you. These fees should reflect costs and profit.

To earn a profit is a basic American freedom, but far too often nurses feel they should provide their services gratis. This is a serious problem in the nursing profession, and it can keep nurses from providing better care to clients.

Another way to generate revenue for your practice is to provide consultation to other nurses seeking advice about private practice. Consultation can take place at your practice or at their home, by appointment. A modest fee (at least $50 per consultation) should be applied in addition to any travel expenses. Creative contracting with clinics, agencies, other private nurse practitioners, or hospitals could be another source of revenue. Experimentation with this could open several new doors for client care.

The National Academy of Science's Institute of Medicine made a study recently on primary health care; it says that nurse practitioner services should not only be covered by public and private health carriers, but also nurses should be reimbursed at the same rate as physicians, for the same services. As yet no third-party payer, such as Medicare or Blue Shield, has analyzed the Institute's equal reimbursement recommendation.[3]

The compensation for the roles we perform should be in line with the responsibility we have for human life, Mauldin explains. Nurses spend the most time with clients. It is the nurse who accurately reports client status and whose judgments and evaluations are most respected. Often the nurse is the only protector the client has.

In all other aspects of health care, cost is no object. Why is this not so when nurses are considered? Nurses are the best health care bargain the public has, and yet nursing lacks the monetary incentives to provide even better nursing care. Nurses want a monetary incentive during these inflationary times to enable them to provide more sophisticated care to the public. Nurses want greater recognition and greater reimbursement for the services they provide.[4]

Although private practice is not meant to be gratuitous, at times nurses can provide gratis care to the needy, indigent client.

Fee Schedules

Creating a fee schedule can be a difficult task. Very few models are available for reference.

Table 11-2, Fee Schedule of Nursing Services, correlates the services in Table 5-1, Schedule of Nursing Services, to meaningful, dignified, and reasonable fees.

Table 11-2 is only a fee guideline. To prepare an inclusive list of services and their fees is not feasible. How you determine your actual fee to the client will depend upon several prevailing factors, which are in a constant state of change. These variables will differ depending upon where your practice is located. Turn to page 153 for a list of some of these factors.

Table 11-2 Fee Schedule of Nursing Services

* Nursing services are usually available on the same day or by appointment.
* Spanish- and English-speaking nurses are available.
* Consultation with your physician and referral are provided as needed.

Fee per office visit (includes counseling and teaching up to one hour)	Services	Contact the office for home visit rates
$20	1. Alcohol counseling	
10–15	2. Drawing blood for laboratory study	
20	3. Bowel and bladder training	
20–25	4. Catheter care: a. Changing, inserting, and removing b. Hygienic care c. Irrigations d. Explaining and teaching	
15–20	5. Child development assessment	
15–20	6. Colostomy care: a. Irrigations b. Dressing or bag changes c. Client and family teaching for home care	
15–25	7. Diabetic care: a. Diet therapy explained b. Insulin therapy c. Personal hygiene d. Exchange diet provided and taught e. Urine testing f. Drawing of blood for laboratory analysis	
20	8. Nutrition counseling (diets explained)	
15–20	9. Drug abuse counseling	
Fee individualized	10. Emergency treatment (limited). Contact your nearest emergency department.	
20	11. Group therapy	

$15–20   12. Histories:
     a. Nursing observations
     b. Nursing diagnosis
     c. Physical and neurological status
     d. Other

20   13. Inhalation therapy:
     a. Teaching
     b. Breathing exercises
     c. Oxygen therapy
     d. Respirator therapy

Fee individualized   14. Injections:
     a. Taught for self-administration where applicable
     b. Given by professional nurses

15–20   15. Drug therapy (prescribed medication):
     a. Counseling
     b. Teaching self-administration
     c. Given by professional nurses

15   16. Irrigations:
     a. Eyes
     b. Ears

Highly individualized   17. Pre- and post-hospital care and counseling

15–20   18. Prenatal counseling and teaching

15–20   19. Postpartum counseling and teaching

20–25
At times individualized   20. Psychosocial counseling:
     a. Crisis intervention
     b. One-to-one relationship
     c. Interviewing, counseling
     d. Referral

15–20   21. Range of motion

15–20   22. Rehabilitation:
     a. Assist
     b. Support
     c. Teach independence
     d. Prosthetic care

10–15   23. Suture removal

15–20	24. Tracheotomy and tracheostomy care: a. Laryngectomy patients
8–12	25. Vision exams: a. Snellen's chart b. Modified Snellen's chart
10–15	26. Vital signs: a. Temperature, pulse, respirations b. Blood pressure c. Management of these
10–15	27. Walker and crutch training
20–25	28. Wound care: a. Cleansing b. Applying dressings and changes c. Teaching personal home care
Highly individualized	29. Stress management
Individualized	30. Hypertension control
Individualized	31. Obesity control
Individualized	32. Counseling provided to school students
15–20	33. Interviewing
0	34. Referral:
Individualized fee with counseling	a. To physicians b. To agencies c. To nurses d. To other health care providers

Unforeseen services that could be provided may be referred. Care and teaching aspects are oriented to allow self home care where appropriate.

Factors To Determine Fee
- amount of time required to perform the procedure
- level of responsibility required in the procedure
- type of procedure itself
- amount of preparation to perform the procedure:
  a. appropriation and preparation of materials
  b. consultation with nurses
  c. consultation with physicians
- amount of self-preparation

- distances traveled and time spent:
  a. to prepare for the procedure
  b. to visit the client at home
- cost of living in your locale and inflation
- maintenance costs
- start-up costs
- profit

It is only fair to apprise your client of your fee before seeing the client. Allow the public to view your fee schedule in your office or explain it over the phone if needed. Quote basic charges only over the phone. Explain to the client that there may be unforeseen additional charges.

To establish the fee for a home visit, consider the distance to be traveled and the time it takes. An additional charge of approximately $7 to $10 may be appropriate for a nearby home visit. Home visits to places far away require individualized rate setting. Clients should be informed to contact the practice for home visit rates.

The cost of equipment is billed as an extra charge to the client. Apprise the client of this also. Thus, clients must pay a fee for nursing service and for health care equipment or supplies. Inform the client that health carriers rarely, if ever, reimburse clients for nursing services, but often reimburse for materials. Also inform your clients that they can deduct your fees on their income taxes. They may recapture some of this money by lowering their taxable income. These facts usually do not hinder your client or case load.

An example of the costs of a catheter change would be:

Home visit with nursing service	$25.00
Catheter	5.00
Catheter kit	7.00
Pack of chux	6.00
Sterile saline	1.00
Drainage bag	2.50
2 syringes	.80
Total	$47.30

Equipment costs	$22.30
Nursing costs	25.00

This nursing care entailed obtaining written orders, consulting with the physician, purchasing equipment (laying out these funds personally before-hand), driving to the client's home 11 miles away, and spending just over one hour providing skilled nursing care to the client and relatives. In this visit a history was obtained, a care plan devised, the procedure performed, the client and relatives were consulted, follow-up care was planned, and results were reported to the physician.

Clients who need the services listed on the Schedule of Nursing Services are in abundance throughout all communities. Nurses practicing from private practices could meet a great deal of clients' needs while they keep the client home in the comfort of familiar surroundings and loved ones. At the same time, the nurses could generate meaningful reimbursement for quality care at a fair and reasonable cost to clients.

Nurses in private practice caring for three clients a day, four days a week, similar to the cited home visit, could produce $300 a week revenue just from these 12 home visits. From this incoming revenue, expenses and profit are extrapolated. Overall, the nurses have the potential to raise their salaries sizably. A regular income of $300 a week amounts to $15,600 a year.

Many of these clients would be revisited periodically. These visits could be set up as community rounds or in-practice visits. You may not believe that many such clients exist, but they do. They are hidden under our noses in nursing homes, physicians' practices, and in other mechanisms of health care delivery. Many of these mechanisms are overcrowded and needlessly keep clients away from the comfort of their homes and loved ones. Nurses can reach out to them via private practice, benefiting the client, public, and the nurses themselves. It enables families to have a family nurse.

Usually physicians are unwilling or unable to make home visits. Even if a physician did make a home visit, the fee would have to be higher and a shorter stay afforded the client. Physicians are too busy to offer this type of service. Nurses should step in and fill these roles while they are available.

Cazalas points out the factors that affect client acceptance of nurse practitioners: the nurse practitioners' personal and unique skills and services, their willingness to consult with the client's physician, and the information the client receives about the nurse practitioners' capabilities, benefits, and services. Clients were as satisfied with nurse practitioners as with physician assistants. Studies demonstrate that clients' satisfaction with nurse practitioners is equal to or greater than their satisfaction with physicians.[5]

A few examples of client care services follow. Note the referrals, services, and billing.

Thomas Ryan: Multiple Sclerosis Patient

Thomas Ryan is 56 years old, 6 feet 2 inches, and 180 pounds. He is confined to bed with multiple sclerosis. He needs a catheter and rides to the Veterans Administration (VA) Hospital by ambulance for routine catheter changes. The VA hospital is 20 miles away; the drive takes about 45 minutes each way. The physician in the hospital told the client about the author's private practice, hoping to save him the trauma of an ambulance ride for routine care. Also, the physician was saving the hospital money by eliminating the payment for ambulance service.

The client contacted the private practice. Needed data and written orders were obtained.

1. Change Foley catheter and irrigate it as necessary.
2. Use Foley catheter 18-5 and increase size to 20-5 when needed.

The home visits cost $25. Vital signs were always taken, records were kept, and the physician was kept informed, as is the case with all clients.

Thomas is doing well, but needs support when depressed. Care of Thomas is ongoing; his needs are met regarding his multiple sclerosis. The client's wife pays the fees. They both realize the benefits they have gained by having their own nurse.

Susan Koster: Diabetic

Susan Koster is an 80-year-old diabetic who also has retinopathy and vascular insufficiency of each leg. She administers her own insulin daily, U. 80, N.P.H., taking 44 units. She is able to do this alone.

The supervising nurse of the local Public Health Department asked me to visit the client daily at 6:00 A.M. to give Vitamin B_{12} injections for a period of eight days. The Public Health Department was unable to provide a nurse in that sequence, so it referred the client to a private nurse practitioner. The supervisor said that the client could not pay for this care but that she definitely needed it.

The client and physician were close to the private practice. The physician gave orders:

1. Examine sites of insulin administration.
2. Give client Vitamin B_{12} intramuscularly (I.M.), 1000 micrograms (mcg.) daily.
3. Supervise insulin administration.
4. Evaluate client's condition.

The client was contacted, and the visits began the next morning. The Public Health Department provided the client with the syringes and vitamins. Home visits were made for four of the eight days. Things were going fine until the fourth day when a bulge on the client's left leg was noticed. It was an enlarging aneurysm, and it needed immediate medical attention. Susan complained of severe pain in this area, and she could hardly walk.

The physician was notified at once and ordered her to the hospital where he performed an aortic bypass and saved the client's leg. I visited her in the hospital and, after discharge, at home. She insisted on paying me $10 for the time I spent with her. Although I refused payment, she insisted, so I accepted it to assuage her feelings of self-worth.

I thanked the supervisor at the Public Health Department, and we submitted a Medicare form, hoping to obtain payment. I requested $40, or $10 per visit. Where the form asks for the physician's signature, I signed and made it clear that a nurse, not a physician, had performed the care and submitted the form for payment. The physician signed alongside. A copy of the physician's orders were sent with the request-for-payment form, but to no avail. The form was returned saying that Medicare cannot pay for nursing care on a fee-for-service basis. Had Medicare paid, the $10 would have been returned.

This client is alive and well today. Notes were maintained, and a copy was sent to the physician. The Public Health Department treats her in conjunction with her physician and my private practice. Further referrals have developed as a result.

Richard Mauro: Paraplegic

Richard Mauro is 23 years old, 5 feet, 11 inches, and weighs 150 pounds. He worked for a local electrical and telephone company until his accident.

He was trimming a tree to allow room for new high power wires to be installed. The tree limb broke, and he fell to the ground, fracturing his right femur and spinal column. The femur and spinal vertebra healed well, but the severed spinal cord did not. He was left a paraplegic with a neurogenic bladder.

The client was referred to the author's private practice a year after the accident by his urologist, who hoped that home visits could be made to change the catheter. The catheter needed to be changed every three days, and the client had to travel 25 miles one way to the urologist.

The client contacted the practice. We called the physician for collaboration. The physician wrote these orders:

1. Change Foley catheter when clogged, as necessary.
2. Catheter may be irrigated daily with water that has been boiled, if needed.
3. Use Foley catheter size 18-5.
4. Keep me informed of progress.
5. Teach client to change catheter by himself.

The home visits were set up for evenings or mornings at $20 each, since there were so many of them, and the client lived nearby. Richard's mother stocked the closet with equipment and paid the nursing fees.

When a change was needed, he would call the practice for a nurse to visit him. If we were out, he would leave a message on the answering machine. Even if he had to wait, it was only a few hours until a nurse arrived. This meant he had to endure only an uncomfortably filled bladder. If it were serious enough, he could visit the emergency department or physician until he learned to change it himself.

Visiting him at home eliminated the transportation trauma and reduced his costs for the physician and ambulance. After a long time, some of his benefits ran out, and he had to begin paying for his services by himself.

The catheter changes and teaching went well. He was disturbed about his body image and sex life. Many hours were spent talking with Richard about these things. Offering time and listening meant a great deal to him. The physician explained that he could have children and sexual relations. This information helped his image and kept him from depression.

He is long since independent of nursing care, and he is doing well. He has a job, a girlfriend, and a car. He may get married soon.

Mrs. Baker: Terminal Cancer Patient

Mrs. Baker was a 74-year-old woman who lived with her husband, 15 miles away from the practice. She was five feet three inches tall and weighed 120 pounds. She and her husband lived in her daughter's home.

The patient had metastasized abdominal cancer and was postoperative from a subtotal gastrectomy in a nearby city hospital. She was recuperating at her daughter's house in the suburbs. A neighbor, a physician in a local emergency department, was visiting her to provide necessary wound care.

Mrs. Baker's wound was healing very slowly, and the physician friend realized that someone would have to attend to wound irrigation and care over a long period of time. The physician discussed the case with the nurses in the emergency department where he was employed to see if they could suggest someone to care for the client. These nurses referred this practice.

The daughter contacted this private practice. Written orders from the neighboring physician were obtained. They were:

1. Home visits.
2. Irrigate abdominal wound with hydrogen peroxide, and dress it with a dry, sterile dressing, daily (O.D.).
3. Vital signs O.D.
4. Regular diet.
5. Out of bed as much as she wants.
6. Continue until wound heals.
7. Client is to bathe one-half hour prior to visit.

The equipment was already in the daughter's home. The fee would be $12 a day since it was daily and would last possibly 40 days. Home visits were to be at 6:00 P.M. from Monday to Friday and on weekends at 10:00 A.M. The bill was to be submitted at the end of the therapy.

The home visits were made, and it was observed that she was becoming weaker. Her vital signs were changing. Her pulse and respiratory rate were steadily rising. The physician was contacted immediately and ordered in writing:

1. Vitamin B_{12} I.M., 1000 mcg. every two weeks.
2. Give oxygen as needed.

This equipment was brought into the home. The daughter was taught how to administer the oxygen and the injection so that when care for the wound was finished, she could provide for her mother.

The client was allergic to aspirin and erythromycin. Luckily, the wound never became infected. It finally healed, and services were terminated.

The patient went home to her native country and town to die. Her husband went with her, as did her daughter. Many, many long sessions were spent in the den with the family discussing the client's future and care. The family needed guidance in coping with the ensuing death of their loved one. That guidance was provided by the nurse practitioner.

Mrs. Baker wrote a lovely letter from her new home. She invited me to visit her there. She also asked me to go home with her as her nurse, but the daughter felt that it would be best if she went so that she could be closer to her mother.

Mary Rogers: Accident Victim

Mary Rogers is 28 years old, has been married for seven years and has no children. She is an unemployed social worker, and her husband works full time as a salesman. She is five feet tall and weighs 120 pounds. She called the office seeking a nurse to make home visits to give her injections for pain. Her physician referred her. Mary suffered a leg injury in an automobile accident and has to take pain medication via injection morning and evening.

The response to her call was positive—the practice would treat her. Over the phone the necessary information was recorded about herself and her physician. The physician and client are local, so a visit was made to the physician to pick up written orders. The orders were:

1. Give Mary Rogers 30 milligrams of Talwin I.M., twice a day, and every 4–6 hours, as necessary.

2. Follow this regimen for one month.
3. Contact me as needed during the month and after the one-month period.

The syringes and Talwin were purchased at a participating drugstore, and the practice was reimbursed by the client.

There was very little problem with treating this client. Medication was primarily needed during the hours when her husband was present.

A history was taken. There was counseling with the client and husband and open communication. They were advised of the cost for the visits beforehand. At least two home visits were required a day, morning and night, and maybe some in between. It was explained that for a treatment of 15 days, regardless of how many visits were made, the cost would be $150. Therefore, if the treatment ran the full 30 days, the cost to the client would be $300. The first few visits took one hour; after that they were about 25 minutes.

The client basically wanted a morning and evening injection. The morning injection enabled her to get through the day, and the evening injection helped her to sleep well. She either received the Talwin at home or had to be hospitalized only for pain medication. She chose to stay at home and do some mild housework, even though her insurance company would not reimburse her for this prescribed fee-for-service, professional nursing care. She received excellent care for a low cost in her home, and she was taught how to properly use crutches and then a cane. She ventilated quite often about her accident, future, and family life. Counseling was provided often.

Vital signs were always recorded, and observations made; all were recorded in nurse's notes filed at the practice. The physician was informed of the client's progress. In 27 days she received a total of 37 injections. The bill to her was $300, and her husband promptly paid it. Mary Rogers is no longer in need of her cane, nursing care, or medical care.

Billing and Collection

Collecting fees is easiest and most appropriate if clients are billed at the time of treatment. Clients should be apprised of your fee, or the basic fee at the time they contact you for care. Thus, when you visit them at home or they visit you in your practice, they are well aware of your fees and are willing to reimburse you accordingly.

Collecting your fees can be a serious problem unless you learn to ask for payment with each visit. You may make a mutual agreement to hold payment until termination of services. Often the problem with paying health care bills is not with clients, but with nurses' squeamishness to discuss fees, bills, and payment with clients. Nurses need to realize that they are worth their fees.

Nurses should feel proud when they bill at an appropriate rate for their unique, professional services. Mauksch has no qualms when it comes to charging an appropriate fee for delivery of quality professional nursing services. The client needs the skilled care that a competent educated nurse can provide. A less-prepared person cannot provide the same care. This is true for all nurses. There are skilled and sophisticated services they can render that others less prepared cannot.[6]

Sometimes clients don't pay their bills for lengthy periods of time. You or your receptionist can ask them nicely to catch up on arrears. Often, clients have several excuses. Calling them a day or two before their next scheduled appointment and asking them to please bring at least partial payment is a good way to stimulate payment. It separates clients who honestly forget from those who purposely do not pay. In cases where your phone calls bring no payment and the client has no good excuse, you need have no compunction about using more drastic collection methods. Collection agencies or small claims courts may be helpful.

A problem with collections is that most people dread asking for payment. Reschke agrees that collection at time of treatment is the most efficient form of payment for you and your clients. There are some steps you can follow to boost the amount of fees clients pay before leaving your practice.

First, if you are aware of the expenses you incur to provide client care, requesting payment is easier. Always request payment or partial payment with a smile and kind, warm tone of voice before the client leaves the office. This practice establishes the custom for clients to pay their bills before leaving the office, and it reduces your billing costs. Further rapport can be established with your client as now you can wish them well and further determine if they comprehend their health regimen.

Some clients will need to be mailed bills, monthly. With these, a personal note requesting payment may prove helpful. A collection agency may need to be utilized, but before doing that, a final call or letter from you requesting payment, informing the client that a collection agency may be employed and that you may terminate the client, may be the jolt the client needs to pay the bill. Try to protect clients' credit ratings, but if they will not pay, use a collection agency.[7]

Termination

Sometimes clients simply cannot afford your fees. For these cases, a sliding scale could be employed for billing. Bill what they can afford, but bill. The reason for this is that in the client's payment of their bill for your service, they gain a sense of pride for being able to pay their way. You are not expected to provide free care to the public either. But on occasion, you could waive payment. You will probably find that doing this from time to time can be exhilarating. To save the client from purchasing equipment, you can use samples or buy it at a discount. You can also refer the client to the Public Health Department. These kinds of clients need not be terminated from your services.

Recalcitrant clients, who refuse to pay even when they can, should be terminated. You need not provide care for them when they disrespect your worth. Remember, though, that some clients may intend to pay you, but they may be slow payers. Your patience with them is the best measure for collection; it's a matter of time for some people.

When a client simply refuses to pay but wishes further service, you have no alternative but to release the client from your care. Send a letter to the client informing him of this. Mail this letter by certified or registered mail, so that you have a return receipt. This will be proof that the client received the letter. Write the account off, and leave the rest to the collection agency.

When terminating clients, Vogl explains that it is best to keep copies of your attempts to reach and inform the client. If clients refuse to claim registered or certified letters, send a mailgram. If this fails, send an ordinary first-class letter. A rule of thumb is that a first-class letter, properly addressed and bearing sufficient postage, is presumed to have been delivered. Have the post office provide you with a certificate of mailing, proving you did mail a letter to the client at said address.

When these methods do not work and the client visits you again, inform the client of termination in front of a witness. You must continue to treat a client for a specific disease process once you have taken responsibility for it. You do not have to take the client back for a new and unrelated condition.[8]

Deductions

Most of your expenses will comprise start-up fees and maintenance fees. You could also add entertainment, which may or may not come under miscellaneous. Entertainment is the cost of entertaining a potential business partner or a consultant, while you are developing professional relations in regard to your practice.

Taxes must be prepared by you or an accountant at each year's end. An accountant should prepare a long form; in this way your practice can enjoy better benefits of claimed expenses. Accountants are useful since they must constantly keep abreast of current tax laws and their applications. The accountant's fees are worth the price as you may regain sizable amounts of revenue spent for expenses.

An accountant will probably be more proficient at preparation of your personal as well as your business' tax forms than you are. This does not mean that you do not understand your tax responsibilities, but does mean that skillful use of an accountant can enable you to gain the benefits from the tax laws more fully. It is helpful if you prepare all of the expenses and receivables for the accountant's use. By working closely with your accountant, you can become further informed of the financial techniques you could apply to benefit your business.

Battersby points out that as the end of the year approaches you should examine how your income and deductions look. If your income is low, you may want to hold off purchasing until the next year. Thus the purchases next year could be used to reduce that year's taxable income. You may wish to itemize deductions and compare them to the standard deduction.

You can deduct business expenses, depreciation of property, education, and travel, meals, and lodging related to education or consultation regarding your profession. Many other expenses are deductible: accountant's fees, interest charges, contributions to charity, dues to professional associations, trade journals, medical expenses, uniforms, cleaning, and much more. Time wisely spent examining your finances and expenses and comparing various ways to prepare your taxes can save you considerable amounts of money.[9]

SUMMARY

You should be able to anticipate the costs that will be incurred from starting and maintaining your own business. This information may help clarify many questions regarding finances as well as real and psychological barriers to conducting a private nursing practice. Physicians have long enjoyed the freedom, luxury, financial rewards, and satisfaction in caring for others that private practice offers. It is time nurses, their clients, and the public benefited by this, too.

No mystery should surround the financial management of a private practice. In the past it may have seemed arcane, but nurses now can benefit by a greater comprehension of this aspect of their profession.

Hopefully, nurses will begin to place greater value on their services. National leaders in the nursing profession must realize this greater value and motivate governmental action to pass these values on to the public by letting the public obtain a greater amount of nursing care through insurance. Practices that have been esoteric to other health care professionals have discriminated against the public and nursing.

NOTES

1. Betty C. Agree, "Beginning an Independent Nursing Practice," *American Journal of Nursing* 74, no. 4 (April 1974): 639.

2. Lawrence I. Subrin, C.P.A., "The Business Aspects of Private Nursing Practice," *Journal of Nursing Administration* 7, no. 7 (September 1977): 51.

3. David W. Sifton, ed., "Nursing News; Study Advocates Equal Pay for Nurse Practitioner and M.D. Doing Same Work," *RN* 41, no. 9 (September 1978):25.

4. Brenda C. Mauldin, R.N., "Professional Work Rates Professional Pay," *RN* 41, no. 9 (September 1978): 43.

5. Mary W. Cazalas, R.N., J.D., *Nursing and the Law* (Germantown, Maryland: Aspen Systems Corporation, 1978), pp. 95–6.

6. Ingeborg G. Mauksch, R.N., "Paradox of Risk Takers," *AORN Journal* 25, no. 7 (June 1977): 1312.

7. Elaine M. Reschke, R.N., "It's Easy to Collect Fees at Time of Treatment," *Physician's Management* 17, no. 7 (July 1977): 9, 10, 13, 14.

8. A. J. Vogl, ed., "Practice Management: If a Certified Termination Letter Isn't Claimed," *Medical Economics* (September 5, 1977), pp. 55–6.

9. Mark E. Battersby "Year-End Tax Savings for Nurses," *Nursing Care* 9, no. 11 (November 1976): 19–20.

Chapter 12

Private Practice and the Law

Mary Williams Cazalas, R.N., J.D.

This chapter provides nurse practitioners with basic information about the law, the workings of the legal system, and the role of each branch of the government in creating, administering, and enforcing the law. Particular emphasis is placed on how the law applies to private nurse practitioners.

GOVERNMENTAL ORGANIZATION AND FUNCTION

The government of the United States is divided into three branches that serve as checks and balances against each other. The legislative branch is responsible for passage of legislation—the constitution, statutes, and regulations. The executive branch is composed of the president and the agencies under his control responsible for assuring compliance with the law. Some enforcement agencies are the Federal Bureau of Investigation, the United States' Attorney's Office, Customs, and the Social Security and Veterans' Administrations. The judicial branch interprets the law; when the language of the law is not clear, the court looks to prior judicial decisions and legislative history to determine legislative intent.

The *common law* of England prevails in England and, by derivation, in most of the United States. It is a system of elementary rules and a general declaration of continually expanding judicial principles. Broadly speaking, it is that great body of unwritten law founded upon general custom, usage, or common consent, and in natural justice, or reason. It is custom long acquiesced to or sanctioned by immemorial use in judicial decisions.[1]

Louisiana follows the *civil law* derived from Spanish, French, and Roman law. The drafters of the Louisiana Civil Code of 1808, which was revised in 1825 and 1870, used the Code Napoleon as a model. Some other states have incorporated civil law principles, e.g., community property; however, most of the law, in states other than Louisiana, is common law.

Cases that involve law of more than one state may result in a conflict of laws. Often, it is difficult to determine which state's law to apply. Our society is controlled by international, federal, and state laws. Cases decided by state and federal courts form a precedent for deciding similar issues in subsequent cases, and, although civil law does not follow precedent, Louisiana courts look to prior decisions for guidance, as do courts in common law states. Cases decided in one state are not binding on the courts of another state, although they may be considered in rendering decisions. In the federal judicial system, one circuit is not bound by the decision of another circuit, but one circuit court may review another circuit court's decision on a particular issue. Circuit courts may decide to overrule prior holdings from their own circuit.

In each state and judicial system, there are lower courts, appellate courts, and a state supreme court. There are city or municipal courts and administrative bodies. The federal court system is composed of district courts, appellate courts, and the U.S. Supreme Court. There are federal administrative bodys and the Federal Court of Customs. Some cases can be taken from the state courts to the U.S. Supreme Court, which is the court of last resort.[2]

A court may have jurisdiction over both civil and criminal actions, or it may be limited to either civil or criminal. The legislative bodies of each state and of the federal government determine the jurisdiction of courts.[3]

A *criminal action* is brought by the state against a defendant charged with violation of a law. The party prosecuted is the defendant. A criminal defendant may be an individual, a corporation, a partnership, or a public entity such as a city, state, or county. A *civil action* is one brought by an individual, corporation, partnership, or state or federal government against an individual, corporation, partnership, or government. A *tort* is a civil wrong and may also be a criminal act, e.g., assault and battery. Civil actions may be brought in contract.[4]

ANATOMY OF A TRIAL

Pleading—Complaint, Answer, Counterclaim, Crossclaim

A trial begins with the filing of a petition or complaint in which the *plaintiff,* the party bringing the suit, sets forth whom is being sued (the *defendant*); the basis for the suit; the amount of damages; and what judgment is being sought. This pleading is served by a sheriff, constable, or federal marshall on the party sued. A defendant, once served, should consult an attorney for legal assistance. Following service, there is a time limit, the *statute of limitation,* within which an answer is to be filed. If no answer is filed, the plaintiff can obtain a default judgment, without notice to the defendant, by proving the allegations in court. A judgment may be rendered in favor of the plaintiff and the right of the defendant to assert defenses to the allegations in the complaint may be lost unless the latter can show good cause—such as lack of service of the complaint —for failure to answer. A defendant has the right to appear before the court on his or her own behalf, but generally, it is better to obtain legal counsel. A person not familiar with the law may not properly present his or her case and justice may not prevail.[5]

Under the Federal Tort Claims Act, a claim is made with the agency the personnel of which the plaintiff alleges committed the act of negligence. At an administrative proceeding, a determination is made as to the merits of the complaint. Administrative remedies must be exhausted prior to filing suit in the federal court. A sovereign entity, such as a state or the federal government, can be sued only if it agrees to be sued and only in the manner in which it agrees to be sued. The procedure is provided by the legislature by statute and the agency may pass regulations to implement the statute. When the federal government is sued, there is no right to a trial by jury. A suit against an individual in a state or federal court may be before a jury, the trier of fact; the judge instructs the jury as to the law. In a trial without a jury, the judge is the trier of fact.

Once the answer is filed, a defendant may also wish to bring an action, or *counter claim,* against the plaintiff. The defendant may allege a cause of action growing out of the same factual situation as that which the plaintiff has alleged in the complaint. In federal court, this is called a *compulsory counter claim* because the claim must be brought in the same action as the plaintiff's suit. A defendant may bring an action against the plaintiff that has arisen from a different set of facts than those alleged in the complaint, which is a *permissible counter claim,* as it could be brought in a separate action. A defendant may file a *cross claim* in order to bring into a suit a codefendant, one the defendant feels is totally or partially liable to the plaintiff for what is alleged in the complaint.[6]

Discovery—Depositions, Interrogatories, Admissions of Fact

The purpose of the law is to determine the truth and arrive at a just disposition of the action. In order to accomplish this, legislative bodies have provided for discovery techniques to determine the facts. *Interrogatories* are lists of questions asked of both parties. *Depositions* are statements taken by questioning the parties and witnesses. Depositions usually are not made before a judge. If a problem arises during the deposition, a judge can be contacted, but this rarely occurs. Depositions of health care providers are usually taken in their offices or in the hospital or attorney's office.[7]

Depositions are used to preserve testimony, as when persons are elderly and there is danger of death prior to trial, or when persons cannot attend the trial. Depositions may be introduced in court in lieu of the witness' testimony, when the witness is not available or if both parties agree. However, it is usually better to have the witness testify before the trier of fact. The witness' credibility usually is more easily ascertained by observation during the trial procedures than by reading a transcript of the testimony. Depositions may be used for impeachment when statements made in court are contradictory to those in the deposition. A request for admission of facts by the parties may be filed. These methods help determine the facts and circumstances and narrow the contested issues, which facilitate the conducting of the trial by reducing the time required for trial and by lessening the cost to the parties. Ancillary or summary proceedings may take place between filing of the suit and the trial on the merits.[8]

The rules of discovery differ among the states and the federal government. Some states have used the federal rules of procedure in drafting their rules. Some do not permit written interrogatories in malpractice or other negligence cases. Some states do not permit oral depositions before a suit is filed, and the depositions may be taken only from those parties involved in the legal action. In other jurisdictions, use of discovery is more liberal. Discovery and disclosure should be used as an opportunity to obtain information. To be properly prepared, the attorney must use discovery to learn the facts and circumstances of the case.[9] Judges may excuse an attorney for not knowing some law or case, but not knowing the facts of one's case is inexcusable.

In a malpractice case, usually the parties involved know the facts and are called on to testify. Oral depositions and interrogatories prior to trial may provide the attorney with sufficient information to assess the likelihood of winning or losing the case and to determine whether, and what, settlement should be made. Generally, discovery should be pursued early in the case, to determine who should be named as a defendant and to avoid not naming a proper defendant. Failure to sue a proper defendant may be legal malpractice if the attorney should have known the proper party and if the statute of limitation runs before suit is filed against that party. Residents and interns may leave a medical facility and be difficult to locate. Early discovery enables the attorney to assess the facts, and, if no cause of action is found, the case can be dismissed.[10]

It is usually stipulated by attorneys that all objections to questions, except to form, will be reserved until the time of trial. Under such a stipulation, the party deposed will be required to answer all questions during examination that do not violate constitutional privilege, without regard to the admissibility of the answer into evidence. When a witness refuses to or is instructed by an attorney not to answer, the deposition can be stopped and an order from the court obtained to compel the witness to answer. Usually, however, attorneys change the form of the question and rarely is it necessary to bring the issue before the court to compel an answer.[11]

Questioning Witnesses

Attorneys of medical personnel at depositions and at trial frequently question whether the witness has reviewed office records and hospital charts;

whether the witness has discussed the case with the witness' attorney; whether the witness' recollection of facts is clear. A witness has a right to discuss to what the witness will testify with the attorneys. The attorneys would be unethical if they told the witness what to say. A witness should admit to discussing the case if this has occurred. These questions prevent a witness' stating at the time of trial that recollection of events at the time was faulty. Questions are asked about the facts involved in the case. A witness should always tell the truth; failure to do so is perjury, since testimony at a deposition or trial is taken under oath. Witnesses who lie may well find themselves in their own trap when they are unable to remember what they have said previously. A witness does not belong to either party and has a right to talk with either attorney or both.

A witness should never lie or mislead the court. However, a witness is not required to go beyond that which is asked in responding to a question. After a question is asked, a witness should always pause a sufficient time so that counsel has an opportunity to object in the event there is a basis for which the answer should not be given. Objections may be raised for reasons such as irrelevancy or immateriality of the response solicited. A response may be hearsay, inadmissible under any of the exceptions to the hearsay rule, or it may be a privileged communication. It usually is advisable to answer what is asked without elaborating. This, however, depends on what one wishes to convey, and sometimes it may be proper legal strategy to elaborate in order to convey information better to the fact finder. Too much elaboration may be harmful to a case. Where there is a disagreement among the medical witnesses and testimony is conflicting, it is for the trier of the facts to determine which, if either, witness is correct. The courtroom is not the place to use as a forum to expound on one's theories. The party calling a witness vouches for the witness' testimony. If the witness testifies differently than expected, the attorney may declare the witness hostile; then the party does not vouch for the testimony.

An example of the wrong way to testify is that of the physician at a spinal cord injury center, who considered the Bricker procedure—routing of the ureters through the abdomen—to be malpractice as performed on a paraplegic client. Medical opinion was divided on the correctness of the procedure. The physician opposing the procedure, a government doctor, was advised that it would be best to answer only what was asked and not to volunteer more. The opposing counsel flattered the physician to win him over. As his ego soared, he brought out his then-unpublished article criticizing the Bricker procedure. This proved most damaging to the government and resulted in the filing of a $2 million malpractice suit, which was ultimately settled. It was necessary to convert the physician to a hostile witness.

The Expert Witness

A *fact witness* is a person who knows something about the facts and circumstances involved in a case. An *expert witness* is one who has superior knowledge and ability in an area and whose testimony, therefore, will be of value to the fact finder—either judge or jury—in arriving at a conclusion as to the truth of what has occurred. It is incumbent upon the plaintiff to prove the allegation of the complaint. Once this burden of proof has been sustained, the burden of proof shifts to the defendant to overcome the plaintiff's proof. Testimony of an expert may be necessary to prove the standard of care with which to compare a defendant's actions.

Persons called as experts should provide counsel with curricula vitae setting forth their educational background, experience, awards received, organizations to which they belong, publications, speaking engagements, and any and all other information which shows their expertise in the area in which they are to be qualified at the time of trial. The expert witness may be accepted as an expert by stipulation of the parties. But, if there is no stipulation of a witness' expertise, the witness must be questioned on his qualifications to prove to the court the superior knowledge that makes him or her an expert in the particular field. The opposing counsel then has an opportunity to cross examine regarding the expert's qualifications. The court has wide discretion in deciding whether to accept a witness as an expert.

The party who called the expert is the first to question him or her in the field of expertise. This is followed by cross-examination from opposing counsel and then redirect examination by the counsel who originally called the expert. Cross-examination of any witness is always limited to the scope of direct examination, and redirect examination is always limited to the scope of cross-examination. A witness who does not understand the question should always ask that the question be repeated. The expert witness usually has testified in a deposition prior to the time of trial. Generally, the attorney does not ask the witness a question without knowing what the answer will be. An illustration of this is the eyewitness who sat in the witness chair with his glasses in a case in his pocket. Thinking his vision was poor, the attorney asked, "How far can you see?" The witness thought for a moment and replied, "Well, I can see the moon."

A witness may be qualified as an expert because of special knowledge, skill, experience, training, or education. Such a witness is permitted to give opinion testimony. The trier of fact decides what weight is to be given to expert testimony. For expert testimony to be admissible, it must deal with a crucial issue and not with collateral matters alone. There is generally no requirement that a particular fact be established by an expert; however, courts may demand expert testimony when the area is difficult for a layperson to understand, such as medicine. The expert may be asked to give opinion testimony based on facts within the expert's own knowledge, or on hypothetical questions setting forth facts supported by the evidence and relating to particular matters upon which the expert testimony is sought, assuming the facts are true for purposes of the opinion. Experts should state the reasons for their opinions. The opinion of the expert must be based upon facts which are either proved or assumed and are sufficient to form a basis for the opinion.[12]

Persons experienced in working with narcotics addicts may be qualified as experts to testify in matters related to addiction. An expert may be called to testify as to brain damage indicated by electroencephalograms; the validity and results of various chemical tests; the physical or mental condition of a client; the treatment and prognosis of a person's condition; the cause of injuries; mental capacity of an individual at some particular time; or the future consequences that can be expected to result from a person's physical or mental condition.[13]

The medical expert may base the opinion testified to upon the teachings of medical science and is not limited to an expression of opinion based solely upon that with which he or she is familiar through direct observation and experience. The court may appoint an expert, which may avoid the problem of having a battle of partisan experts. Testimony of the medical expert must be presented to the trier of fact in an understandable way, which is sometimes difficult because of the specialized and complex subject matter discussed. The hospital record, the physicians' reports, scientific records, charts, graphs, and anatomical models may all be used by the expert, and some or all of these may be introduced into evidence. The treating physician, as well as a nontreating physician to whom a client may be sent for the purpose of an examination with litigation contemplated, may be called upon as fact witnesses and may also be qualified as expert witnesses.[14]

MEDICAL RECORDS AS EVIDENCE

Medical Records in Legal Proceedings

The increasing incidence of personal injury suits and the expanding acceptance of life, accident, and health insurance have made medical records important evidence in legal proceedings. These records aid police investigations, provide information for determining the cause of death, indicate the extent of injury in workmen's compensation or personal injury proceedings, and aid in determining mental competency in civil and criminal cases.[15]

The medical record should be a complete, accurate, up-to-date report of the medical history, condition, and treatment of a client and the result of the hospitalization of the client. A medical record is composed of at least two distinct parts. The first usually is compiled at admission and details the pertinent data of the client's history, e.g., name, age, and reason for admission. The second part is the clinical record, a continuing history of the treatment rendered the client while hospitalized. The information that must be included in this part is prescribed by state licensing rules and regulations. Usually, it must contain the client's physical history, complaints, temperature chart, admitting diagnosis, later diagnoses, consultations, medical notes, laboratory reports of tests, x-ray readings, surgical or delivery records (including anesthesia reports, operative procedures, and findings), nurses' notes, summaries, condition of the patient at the time of discharge, or autopsy findings if deceased, etc. This record is maintained continually by the physicians and nurses who attend the client. In most states, both physicians and nurses must sign or initial the record. All licensing regulations stipulate that all records must be accurate and complete.[16]

Witnesses are permitted to refresh their recollection of facts and circumstances by reviewing medical records. A medical witness who has treated many clients may find it difficult to remember all the facts and circumstances related to a particular client or incident without reviewing the medical records. Lapse of time can dull the memory of some people. A medical record may be admitted as evidence in legal proceedings if the court is assured that the information contained therein is accurate, that it was recorded at the time the event occurred, and that it was not recorded in anticipation of the particular legal proceeding. When a medical record is introduced, its custodian, usually the medical record librarian, must testify as to the manner in which the record was made and the way in which it is protected from unauthorized handling and change. Whether records and other documents are admitted or excluded is governed by the rules of evidence that have been established to assure that the information to be introduced is trustworthy. The court must be convinced that the record is complete, accurate, and timely.[17]

The method of obtaining medical records before trial for discovery purposes and at the time of trial for introduction into evidence is provided by state and federal statutes. A client may consent to the medical records being provided to the party requesting them. If a client refuses to consent, records may be obtained with a court order by filing a *subpoena duces tecum.* If a party or medical care provider refuses to provide the records, a motion or rule to show cause why they should not be provided may be filed and a hearing before a judge held. The judge determines whether the records should be provided and issues an order accordingly. Parties may stipulate that the records may be introduced into evidence. The judge determines admissibility according to the rules of evidence. The best-evidence rule is followed by the court, and the best evidence of a medical record is the original record. The party may make a motion after introduction of the original record that it be substituted with a copy for filing in the court so that the original record can be returned to the custodian, the one who is responsible for maintaining the records.[18]

If an original record cannot be found but a copy is available, the copy may be introduced if there is proof that it is a true copy and the reason that the original cannot be located is proved to the court. A medical record is the property of the health care provider; however, the client has a property right to the information contained in the record and must be given access to this information. The procedure for obtaining access to the record is controlled by statutes in each state. If a health care provider fails to honor a subpoena for a medical record, the court may hold the provider in contempt of court and impose a fine and/or prison sentence.[19]

Under certain circumstances medical records may not be admitted into evidence because of confidential communications between the client and physician that are protected from disclosure. The physician-client privilege may be extended in some states to the nurse-client relationship. The confidentiality of communications in medical situations is a principal tenet of the nursing code of professional ethics. There are also state statutes that forbid physicians, dentists, and other health practitioners from disclosing, without the client's consent, any information acquired during the course of caring for a client. Some of the statutes expressly include disclosures made to professional, registered, or trained nurses, which means that nurses cannot be forced to testify in legal proceedings about information obtained while caring for a client. However, according to most state statutes, nurses are not subject to the restrictions concerning revelation of confidential communications. The courts of a few states have held that, by implication, these statutes include nurses who are assisting or acting under the direction of a physician treating the client.[20] In effect, the physician-patient privilege is extended to nurses as well.

The common law does not recognize a physician-client privilege. However, there was a disposition to recognize a confidential communication between a psychotherapist and a client. Federal Rules of Evidence, 504, does provide for a physician-client privilege when the physician is a psychotherapist. The legislation recognized that in order to obtain benefit from treatment, the client must be willing and able to talk freely. Lack of privileged communication could be detrimental to treatment.[21]

Volume 42 of the *Code of Federal Regulations,* Sections 2.1 through 2.67-1, sets forth what information may be disclosed, to whom it may be disclosed, and the procedure for disclosing information relative to clients receiving treatment for drug abuse in federally funded programs. In this regard, the regulations provide a civil penalty of $500 for the first wrongful disclosure and $5,000 for the second.

Although the statutory protection of information obtained in physician-client relationships applies only to courtroom testimony, there is a general belief that some protection should be afforded the personal and private revelations of clients to physicians to prevent their general dissemination. Physicians do have an ethical duty not to disclose information received from clients. In most states, protection is limited to information furnished the physician that is necessary to enable treatment of the client, and legislation often limits the physician-client privilege to certain kinds of legal actions. Protection may cover information in hospital records as well as communications to physicians. To a lesser extent, these principles also apply to nurses working directly under physicians.[22]

In the operation of a hospital and the delivery of client care, staff physicians and hospital personnel may require the use of information from the records. Moreover, physicians, residents, interns, nurses, and other personnel may consult records for the purposes of research, statistical evaluation, and education. However, if the information so obtained is not kept confidential, the hospital may be held liable.[23]

If the information from medical records is disclosed without a court order or statutory authority to do so and without the client's consent, the hospital or its employees may be held for damages if the client's interests are harmed. Clients have alleged injury in these situations on the grounds of defamation or invasion of their right to privacy.[24]

The restriction on disclosing information obtained in a confidential relationship usually does not apply to criminal matters such as attempted suicide or the unlawful dispensing or taking of narcotic drugs. Likewise, a client may waive the privilege by actions or words. For example, a client who testifies about an illness can no longer claim protection for the information. In addition, some statutes provide that by bringing an action for damages in a personal injury or workmen's compensation claim, the client waives the claim to a privileged communication.[25]

Indiscriminate release of medical records may be considered an invasion of privacy or privilege. The medical care provider that owns the records is entitled to an authorization to inspect and make copies that is signed and acknowledged by the patient or other responsible person. Generally, the attorney should obtain the entire record; a copy of the record should be provided to the expert and fact witnesses for their review before testifying. Oftentimes, the key to the case is found in some part of the record on its review in preparation for trial. The progress notes, physicians' orders, and admit and discharge notes are usually the portions of the record that best reflect the course of the client's hospitalization. The physicians' orders, laboratory and x-ray reports, and temperature records often may be of particular relevance. If records are changed or portions are missing, doubt may be raised as to the verity of the record. The hospital record is of extreme importance in determining the facts in a malpractice or personal injury case.[26]

If a hospital refuses to permit a record to be examined and copied when properly authorized to do so, a lawsuit against the hospital may result in those states where access to medical records cannot be compelled by the court until after a lawsuit is filed. Therefore, it may be wise to permit copying of the record when properly authorized to do so. The nurses' notes may be significant in proof of pain and suffering. The amounts of sedative, narcotic, and analgesic drugs administered to a client and the description of the client's appearance and complaints may well establish the degree of pain and suffering and also mental competency of the client. The information sought from review of the record and from questioning of the witnesses may determine what injury occurred and the extent thereof, the cause of the injury, and whether it was caused by negligence.[27]

The proper party to be sued as causing the injury must be determined and, when there is doubt, all parties who may possibly be responsible for the injury should be sued. If the attorney fails to include a party as a defendant who should have been included, and the statute of limitation passes with the cause of action against that party prescribed, then the attorney may be found guilty of legal malpractice and liable in damages.[28]

Hospital records that conform to the qualifications imposed by the Federal Business Records Act are admissible, although they are hearsay. They may be used to prove such facts as a previous medical condition, condition found at autopsy, prior medical history, a client's subjective and objective symptoms, diagnosis, and treatment. Statements in hospital records that are admissible under the Federal Business Records Act are limited to statements of fact. Hospital records and charts that show a client's condition, medicines administered, etc., are hearsay. They are not admissible into evidence unless they are subject to one of the many exceptions to the hearsay rule or are admissible under some other rule. They may be used to cross-examine a witness who made them or to prove an admission of a party contained in the record. They may be used to refresh present recollection and as past recollection recorded.[29]

A proper foundation must be laid for introduction of medical records. A *subpoena duces tecum* is usually issued to the custodian of the medical records. A foundation is laid through testimony of the custodian to establish trustworthiness of the record in order to admit the record under the Uniform Business Records Act.

STATEMENTS AND AFFIDAVITS

Evidence is admissible when offered to prove that a statement was made or a conversation was had rather than the truth of what was said. Objections to hearsay should be made at the earliest possible moment so that the objection comes before the answer. The jury can be instructed to disregard an answer considered to be hearsay; however, once the jury has heard the statement, it is difficult to disregard it. For this reason, the witness should pause sufficiently after a question to permit counsel to object.

An affidavit is a written statement sworn to before an officer authorized to take oaths, such as a notary public. An affidavit offered into evidence for the truth of any of the allegations it contains is hearsay even though the statements are made under oath. Statements made under oath generally are considered to be trustworthy because of the threat of a perjury conviction if what is contained within is false. Affidavits are accorded considerable dignity and weight although they generally are not admissible into evidence.

Statements or declarations of intent, knowledge, and the state of mind, emotion, sensation, or physical condition are exceptions to the hearsay rule. When the state of mind of a person at a particular time is relevant, declarations made at that time are admissible. When physical condition is relevant to a case, usual and natural expressions and exclamations of a person that are spontaneous manifestations of pain and naturally flow from suffering are competent and original evidence regardless of to whom they are uttered. They may be testified to by any person who has heard them. Statements of medical diagnosis or treatment in describing the medical history, past or present symptoms, pain or sensations, or general character of a cause or external source thereof, insofar as reasonably pertinent to diagnosis and treatment, are not excluded by the hearsay rule even though the declarant is available as a witness.[30]

THE ADVERSARY SYSTEM

The adversary system provides for adjudication of disputes by rules of substantive, evidentiary, and procedural law. An advocate, by zealous preparation and presentation of facts and law, enables the judge and jury to come to the trial with open and neutral minds and render an impartial judgment. The duties of an attorney to the client and to the legal system are the same. The attorney must represent the client zealously within the bounds of the law. Procedures that govern the presentation of the client's position are prescribed largely by legislative enactments, court rules and decisions, and administrative rules.[31]

To assure that justice prevails, the judicial tribunal should be informed and impartial. A civil adjudicative process is designed to promote settlement of disputes. The criminal process is designed to protect society as a whole. When judicial process is abused, the public loses confidence in the legal system. Judicial proceedings should be conducted with dignity and order designed to protect the rights of all parties, avoid undue solicitude for convenience of the judge or jury, and avoid any other conduct calculated to gain special consideration. In adversary proceedings clients are litigants and ill feeling may exist between them, but ill feeling should not influence the attorney.[32]

An attorney should be courteous to opposing counsel and agree to reasonable requests regarding court proceedings, settings, continuances, waiver of procedural formalities and similar matters that do not prejudice rights of the client. The customs of courtesy or practice should be followed unless timely notice is given opposing counsel of the intention not to do so; the attorney should always be punctual. The function of the adversary system depends on cooperation between attorneys and tribunals in utilizing procedures to preserve impartiality of tribunals and make the decisional process prompt and just without impinging on the obligation of attorneys to represent their clients zealously within the framework of the law.[33]

Caution must be used in selecting a competent and ethical attorney. Conduct of attorneys is controlled by the canons of ethics of the Bar Association and the courts. An attorney is required to represent a client zealously within the bounds of the law. An attorney has a duty to both the client and the legal system. Each member of our society has the right to have his or her conduct judged and regulated in accordance with the law; to seek any lawful objective through legally permissible means; and to present for adjudication any lawful claim, issue, or defense. An attorney is not justified in asserting a position in frivolous litigation.[34]

The responsibility of a public prosecutor differs from that of the usual advocate. The prosecutor must seek justice, not merely conviction. This special duty exists because the prosecutor represents the sovereign and, therefore, should show restraint in the discretionary exercise of governmental powers such as selection of cases to prosecute. The accused is to be given the benefit of all reasonable doubt, but the prosecutor has responsibilities different from those of an attorney in private practice. The prosecutor should make timely disclosure to the defense of available evidence known to him which tends to negate the guilt of the accused, mitigate the degree of the offense, or reduce the punishment. Further, a prosecutor should not intentionally avoid pursuit of evidence merely because of the belief that it will damage the prosecution's case or aid the accused.[35]

A government attorney with discretionary powers as to litigation should not continue litigation which is obviously unfair. A government attorney in a civil action or administrative proceeding must seek justice and develop a full and fair record. Position and economic power of the government should not be used to harass parties to bring about unjust settlements or results.[36]

The obligation of loyalty to a client applies to the attorney in the discharge of professional duties only and does not imply an obligation to adopt a personal viewpoint favorable to the client's interest or desires. The attorney must always act so as not to adversely affect the rights of a client in a matter being handled by that attorney and act in a manner that is consistent with the best interest of the client. However, if action in the best interest of the client appears to be unjust, the attorney may ask the client to forego such action. Although the attorney is to represent the client with zeal, there is an obligation to be considerate of all persons involved in the legal process and avoid infliction of needless harm.[37]

Pretrial

Prior to trial, motions may be filed. A motion to compel answers to interrogatories may be filed if answers are insufficient or if a party refuses to answer. A motion may be filed to compel a witness to testify at a deposition. A motion to dismiss the case may be filed when the suit is filed after the statutory time limit for filing has passed, that is, after the statute of limitation has run. Failure to file on time is one of the most frequent reasons for filing a legal malpractice suit. Lack of jurisdiction of the court over the subject matter or over the parties is another basis for dismissal.

A motion for summary judgment is permitted when there are no material facts in dispute and when, as a matter of law, a party is entitled to a judgment. This motion is rarely successful in tort cases, and particularly in medical malpractice actions, because usually there are material facts in dispute. A summary judgment was granted, for example, in a medical malpractice case in which the colon was perforated during a proctoscopic examination and taking of a biopsy. Testimony of the physician who performed the examination and the supervising physician was that they had used all care of the ordinary physician and that this could happen to even the most expert physician. The testimony of the physician called by the patient as an expert witness corroborated the testimony of the treating physicians. The pathology report showed the tissue in the area of the biopsy to be diseased and easily perforated. No material facts were in dispute. Based on this, the judge granted a summary judgment in favor of the defendant physicians.

Pretrial conferences are held with the judge or a magistrate at which an effort is made to narrow the issues in order to conserve time if the case is tried. These conferences also provide an opportunity for negotiation of settlements under the guidance of an impartial party—the judge.

The Trial

If no settlement is reached, the case is set for trial. The first step in the trial, if a jury is not waived, is to select the jury. A right to trial by jury is guaranteed by the Constitution. The procedure of selecting a jury varies, but the procedure used must result in a jury selected from a cross section of the entire community. Jury selection is an art. In selecting a jury, questions are asked sometimes by the judge and sometimes by counsel, depending on the system used by the particular court, to determine whether a prospective juror should be excused for cause by the court. The attorneys also have a designated number of challenges, giving them the right to excuse jurors for any or no reason.

Following jury selection, the plaintiff's counsel makes an opening statement in which what is intended to be proved is told to the court. The opening statement should be presented in an orderly fashion as if telling a story, a preview of what is to be disclosed during the trial through introduction of exhibits and testimony of witnesses. Following the opening statement by plaintiff's counsel, the defense has an opportunity to make an opening statement in order to give the defendant's version of what the trial will unfold. The attorneys for the parties are permitted to state only the facts. When the opening statements are completed, the plaintiff's case is presented. At the close of the plaintiff's case, the defendant may ask for a directed verdict in favor of the defendant if a civil case, or a judgment of acquittal if a criminal case. If this motion is denied, the defendant's case is then presented.

At the close of the defendant's case, another motion for a directed verdict in a civil case or judgment of acquittal in a criminal case may be made by the defendant. If this is not granted, counsel for the plaintiff then gives a closing argument, in which a review of the facts as unfolded by the evidence is presented to the jury. This is followed by the closing argument of the defense counsel, in which the defendant's version of the facts based on the evidence presented is stated. The jury is then charged by the judge as to the law to be applied. The jury retires to the jury room, where it deliberates and attempts to arrive at a verdict. If questions arise that need to be answered, the jury may send their questions out to the judge and the judge may send back a written response, or bring the jury back into the courtroom with both sides present, when a further charge may be given. After the verdict is rendered by the jury, the judgment of the court is handed down, in accordance with the jury's verdict. If the judge disagrees with the jury, a judgment notwithstanding the verdict may be rendered in a civil case. In a criminal case a judgment of acquittal would be rendered.

The losing party can take an appeal to a higher court. The one who appeals is the appellant and the respondent is the appellee. The appellate court is bound by the record that is made in the district court, and no new evidence may be introduced in the appellate court. Therefore, it is crucial that the record be made at the time of trial in the district court. If there is serious doubt as to whether evidence should be introduced and the case is strong without that evidence, it is best to leave it out rather than risk reversal on appeal. If the evidence is crucial, then there is no choice but to attempt to have the evidence admitted in the district court and chance a reversal on appeal.

The trial is transcribed by the court reporter, who is responsible for lodging the record in the appellate court. The party who takes the appeal must write a brief in which the issues to be raised on appeal will be enumerated. A summary of the facts is given, each statement supported with a transcript page so that the court will be aided in verifying statements made and in finding sections of the transcript referred to in the statement of facts. In the argument portion of the brief, each issue is stated with a discussion of why the appellate court should decide in favor of the particular party. The brief should include in the conclusion the relief sought from the appellate court. The brief is filed in the court of appeals and is served on the opposing party or counsel for the opposing party.

The appellee has a specified time in which to file the brief in opposition to the appellant's brief. The appellee's brief should restate the facts and never adopt the facts of the appellant's brief. If the facts of the appellant's brief are adopted, the court may look in the appellant's brief to review the facts, and psychologically this may reinforce the appellant's argument to the detriment of the appellee. The appellee must present a legal argument for each of the issues raised by the appellant, explaining why the appellant's argument is incorrect and why the judgment of the district court should be affirmed. The court of appeals reviews the record and the brief. In some jurisdictions, state and federal, the cases are set for summary calendar without oral argument, or are set for oral argument.

At oral argument, the appellant argues first, the appellee second, and the appellant may reserve some time to present a rebuttal argument. The appellate judges sit in a panel, usually of three, and one of the judges writes the opinion. If the other judges agree, they may or may not write a concurring opinion. If a judge disagrees with the decision of the majority, that judge may write a dissenting opinion. The judgment of the court is the holding in the case and forms a precedent for future cases.

Reasoning expressed in the various opinions is referred to as *dicta* and is not binding on the court in future decisions, but may be helpful in deciding future cases. If a court wishes to decide a case differently from a precedent case, the court may sit *en banc,* that is, all members of the court sitting at the same time, with a majority needed if the holding of a prior decision is not to be followed.

After the appellate court renders its decision, the losing party may apply for a *writ of certiorari* or take an appeal, as the rules provide, to the supreme court, which is the court of last resort. A higher court may affirm the lower court, remand the case for a new trial, or reverse in whole or in part the decision of the lower court. Once the decision is final, the judgment can be executed. If a money judgment is granted, the party must be paid. A defendant may enter bankruptcy, although it will mean loss of assets, in accordance with the provisions of the Bankruptcy Statute. Persons living in states having community property law are subject to the laws of community property, even though the property was accumulated principally from the efforts of the other spouse who is not being sued. Malpractice insurance, which pays for the cost of litigation, including court costs and attorneys' fees, and pays any judgment rendered up to the maximum limits of the policy, is essential. With the large awards made today by the courts, the malpractice coverage must be an adequate amount.

TORTS—CIVIL WRONGS

Medical malpractice has become a crisis in our society. Health care providers find it necessary to practice defensive medicine in anticipation of the filing of a lawsuit against them; this increases the costs of medical care. A malpractice suit has been described as an occupational hazard for the practicing physician. Reasons for the malpractice crisis are a greater awareness of the public about medical care, advances in medical treatment, patients' expectation of results greater than is medically possible, an impersonal attitude of the medical profession towards patients, and the high cost of medical care.

Negligence[38]

Usually medical malpractice suits are filed to recover damages allegedly sustained from negligence. Negligent conduct is that which falls below the standard established by law for protection of others against reasonably greater risk of harm. The majority view considers failure to use the care required under the circumstances to be negligence. Some states recognize the doctrine of degrees of negligence. Slight negligence is failure to use great care; ordinary negligence is failure to use ordinary care; gross negligence is failure to use slight care and borders on willful and intentional conduct. Just as the nursing profession has "Ms. Chase," the legal profession has "the reasonable person." The standard for determining whether conduct of a nurse practitioner was negligent is that of a reasonable nurse practitioner under the circumstances. The nurse practitioner must act like the reasonably prudent nurse practitioner. If the action is reasonable, the nurse practitioner is not negligent and cannot be held liable for any injury that occurs.

What the reasonable nurse practitioner would do under the circumstances is determined by testimony from expert witnesses familiar with the knowledge, duties, and responsibilities of nurse practitioners. Textbooks, medical publications, licensing requirements, and manuals for nurse practitioners provide evidence of what is expected of the reasonable nurse practitioner.

For a person to be liable in negligence, there must have been a duty to conform to a particular standard of conduct for the protection of others from unreasonable risk of harm, a failure to conform to this standard, a causal connection between the conduct and injury sustained, and actual loss or damage. Nominal damages and punitive damages are awarded in some cases. Some states, such as Louisiana, do not award punitive damages.

Where there is no duty for a nurse practitioner to undertake treatment of a client, but treatment is undertaken, the nurse practitioner must then treat the client by exercise of reasonable care. An example is the nurse practitioner who is an expert in treatment of cardiac patients, who observes a person having a heart attack on a downtown street. The nurse practitioner has no duty to undertake treatment of that person. However, if treatment is undertaken, then reasonable care must be exercised in rendering treatment and the care must continue until the client has someone else to render treatment or treatment is no longer necessary.

If a hospital has an emergency room and holds itself out to the public as rendering emergency treatment, nurse practitioners working in that emergency room or taking calls who refuse to treat a client because of inability to pay could be held liable for resulting damages caused by failure to treat, since a duty to undertake treatment could be found under this circumstance.

The community standard in determining what is reasonable care is followed in some jurisdictions. However, there is a trend away from a community standard and towards establishment of a national standard since medical treatment is comparable throughout the United States. Another reason for this change is the difficulty of obtaining testimony of one medical expert against another in the same community. A physician from another locality may be more willing to testify against a member of the medical profession.

Respondeat superior[39] is the term for a form of vicarious liability wherein an employer is held liable for the wrongful acts of an employee even though the employer's conduct may be without fault. Liability predicated on *respondeat superior* may be imposed on an employer only if a master–servant relationship exists between the employer and employee and if the wrongful act of the employee occurs within the scope of employment.

If the employer has the right to control the physical conduct of the employee's performance of duties, then a master–servant relationship sufficient to invoke the doctrine of *respondeat superior* exists. An act is "within the scope of employment" when it is so closely related to what the employee has been hired to do, or so fairly and reasonably incidental to employment, that it may be regarded as a method of carrying out the orders of the employer. Furthermore, the propriety or impropriety of that method has no bearing whatsoever on the determination of whether the act is within the scope of employment.

The doctrine of *respondeat superior* does not absolve the employee of liability for wrongful acts. Not only may the injured party sue the employee directly, but the employer may also seek compensation from the employee for the financial loss occasioned by the employee's wrongful act.

The doctrine of *respondeat superior* does not apply to the wrongful conduct of an independent contractor. An independent contractor is usually an agent of a principal over whom the principal has no right of control concerning the manner in which the work is to be performed. Thus, a master–servant relationship does not exist and, therefore, the doctrine of *respondeat superior* does not apply.

Res ipsa loquitur[40] means "the thing speaks for itself." To apply the doctrine of *res ipsa loquitur,* the following criteria must be present:

1. The injury must be one which usually does not occur in the absence of negligence.
2. The injury must have occurred through an instrumentality or agency that is under the exclusive possession or control of the defendant.
3. The injury must not have been the result of the plaintiff's contributory negligence or assumption of risk.

Sometimes courts have held that the evidence explaining the cause of the injury should be more accessible to the defendant than to the plaintiff. The physician in a malpractice case is usually more able to explain what has occurred. The physician usually has control of the instrumentalities, e.g., surgical instruments and medications, which cause the injury. There is also a growing recognition within the law of a special obligation and duty between a doctor and the patient. The dependent party must be protected from unexplained injury at the hands of one in whom the patient has reposed a trust.

DEFENSES TO ALLEGATIONS OF NEGLIGENCE[41]

Contributory Negligence

Once the plaintiff has established that a defendant has been negligent, the defendant may raise defenses to the claim for damages. The most common defense in a negligence action is contributory negligence, which, when established, constitutes a complete barrier to the plaintiff's damage claim.

When contributory negligence is raised, the defendant claims the conduct of the injured person to be below the standard of care that a reasonably prudent person would exercise for his or her own safety. The elements of contributory negligence are: (1) that the plaintiff's conduct is below the required standard of care; and (2) that there is a connection between the plaintiff's careless conduct and the injury. The defendant contends the plaintiff contributed to the plaintiff's injury.

The rationale for contributory negligence is based on the principle that people must be both careful and responsible for their acts. The plaintiff is required to conform to the same broad standard of conduct, that of the reasonable person of ordinary prudence under like circumstances, and the plaintiff's negligence will be determined and governed by the same tests and rules as the negligence of the defendant. Contributory negligence is a defense to negligence only, and it is not a defense to an intentional wrong to inflict harm.

Comparative Negligence

Comparative negligence is recognized only in a few states. This doctrine provides that where both parties have been found to be negligent or careless, the degree of negligence or carelessness of each party be determined by the trier of fact. Each party is held to be responsible for an appropriate proportion of the injuries. For example, where a plaintiff suffers injuries of $10,000 from an accident, and the plaintiff is found to have been 20 percent negligent, the defendant would be required to pay only 80 percent, or $8,000.

Assumption of Risk

The second most commonly used defense is assumption of risk. This defense simply means that the plaintiff has expressly given consent in advance, thereby relieving the defendant of an obligation of conduct toward the plaintiff and taking the chances of injury from a known risk arising from the defendant's conduct. For example, a private duty nurse who agreed to care for a client with a communicable disease and who contracted the disease would not be entitled to sue the former client for loss of earnings. In taking the job, the nurse agreed to assume the risk of infection and thereby released the client from all legal obligations.

Unavoidable Accident

The defense of an unavoidable accident may be raised where an injury has occurred but the elements necessary to constitute negligence are not present. If a patient's ankle turns and *only* this causes the patient to fall in the hospital corridor, the hospital would not be liable where elements of negligence are absent.

STATUTE OF LIMITATION

The statute of limitation is "a statute prescribing limitations to the right of action on certain described causes of action." No suit can be maintained on such causes of action unless brought within a specified period after the incident occurred. The correct legal terminology is that "the statute of limitation has run."

Whether a suit for personal injury can be brought against a nurse often depends on whether the suit has commenced within a time specified by the applicable statute of limitation. Generally, the statutory period begins when an injury occurs, although in some cases (usually involving foreign objects left in the body during surgery), the statutory period commences when the injured person discovers, or should have discovered, the injury.

There are many technical rules associated with statutes of limitation. Statutes in each state prescribe that malpractice and other personal injury suits must be brought within fixed periods of time, but court decisions and specific statutes in many states have extended the limitation periods substantially. For example, the fact that the injured person is a minor or is otherwise under a legal disability may, under the laws of many states, extend the period within which an action for injury may be brought.

Actions for malpractice may be brought in tort or in contract. A tort is a civil wrong that includes negligence. Most malpractice actions are in tort, as the amount of damages is greater. The plaintiff would not be able to obtain a judgment awarding pain and suffering if the suit were in contract. However, since a contractual relationship does exist, a suit may be brought for breach of contract. If the statute of limitation has run for bringing an action in tort, but not for a suit in contract, the action can be brought in contract.

Some states have passed special statutes setting statutes of limitation or prescriptive periods for bringing malpractice suits. In 1975 Louisiana added a new statute, LA R.S. 9:5628, which provides that no action for damages arising out of patient care brought against any physician, dentist, or hospital licensed under Louisiana laws shall be brought unless filed within one year from the date of discovery of the alleged act, omission, or neglect, provided, however, that claims are filed, at the latest, within a period of three years from the date of the alleged act, omission, or neglect. In Louisiana, tort actions not based on malpractice must be brought within one year from discovery and actions in contract within ten years from the breach of the contract. This statute places a maximum of three years from the act that suit can be brought. Nurses are not included in this act. However, suits brought against parties named in the act are frequently based on alleged malpractice by nurses who are employees of these parties. Therefore, the act indirectly applies to nurses. Nurses may wish to bring before legislatures the necessity of including nurses in legislation involving medical malpractice.

INTENTIONAL WRONGS[42]

Assault and Battery

An assault is an intentional act designed to place another person in apprehension of a battery. A battery is an intentional, unconsented touching of another's person. Liability for these wrongs is based on the right to be free from invasion of one's person.

Clients have sued for assault and/or battery when medical and/or surgical treatment has been rendered without informed consent.

Invasion of Privacy

The right of privacy is the right to be left alone and to be free from unwarranted publicity and exposure to public view. Hospitals, nurses, and physicians may become liable for divulging information about a client to an improper source or for committing unwarranted intrusions into the client's personal affairs.

Defamation

Defamation is a written or oral communication to someone other than the person defamed, concerning a living person, which tends to injure that person's reputation. Libel is written, and proof of damages is not necessary to be actionable. Slander is oral, and actual damages must be proved.

Malicious Prosecution and Abuse of Process

One suing for malicious prosecution or abuse of process must prove perversion of legal process to improper ends. Elements are that the defendant brought an action against the plaintiff, the proceeding was terminated in favor of the party sued, probable cause for the proceeding was absent, and the defendant brought the action because of malice.

CONSENT[43]

Consent may be either oral or written, unless statutory provisions of a particular state provide otherwise. A written consent provides visible proof of consent, whereas oral consent is more difficult to prove. A valid written consent must be signed and must show that the procedure performed was the one consented to and that the consenting person understood the nature of the procedure, the risk involved, and the probable consequences.

General consent forms permitting medical care providers to perform any medical or surgical procedure believed in the client's best interest do not constitute valid consent. Only one who is knowledgeable about the medical or surgical treatment to be rendered should obtain the consent from the client. Generally, the physician should inform the client, as it is the physician who knows best what is to be done. The consent form should be witnessed, and the witnesses selected should be persons who can later be located should litigation be commenced.

Generally, a client's consent is required before treatment is administered. When a client is physically unable or legally incompetent to consent, and no emergency exists, consent must be obtained from a person who is legally authorized to consent on the client's behalf. The person who gives consent for treatment of another must have sufficient information to make an intelligent judgment and must be aware of the risk involved in the procedure. If a procedure needs to be done, and there is doubt as to who has authority to consent and the client is unable to consent, it is always advisable to obtain a court order for protection of the health care provider.

In *In re Osborn,* 294, F.2d 372 (D.C. App. 1972), factors for consideration in determining whether to compel medical care rejected by a client on religious grounds were stated to be whether the client validly and knowingly rejected the medical care and whether there is a sufficient state interest to override the individual's desire based on religious beliefs. The degree of state interest must be compelling.

In determining whether a minor can consent to treatment, the health care provider should look to the statutory law within the state. Some state statutes provide that minors can consent to medical treatment. Courts have also used as a point of reference the requirement of an adult's assent in order to make a minor's obligation binding in commercial matters. As a general proposition, courts have usually held that consent of a minor to medical or surgical treatment is ineffective, and the physician must secure the consent of the minor's parent or someone standing *in loco parentis,* or risk liability. Some courts have held consent of a minor to be sufficient authorization for treatment under certain conditions. Courts have held that minors who are married and emancipated do not require parental consent. Some states have special statutory provisions granting a minor the right to consent to treatment for drug abuse, pregnancy, venereal disease, and medical/surgical care. The safest course to follow is to obtain consent of the minor and also that of the parent, guardian, or spouse. If in doubt, obtain a court order.

Persons who are mentally incompetent have been considered unable legally to consent to medical or surgical treatment. For a person who has been declared legally incompetent by a judicial proceeding, consent of the patient's legal guardian must be obtained. Where no legal guardian is available, a court that handles such matters must be asked to permit the procedure. Equal protection of the law, guaranteed by the Constitution of the United States, may be abridged if a person who is mentally ill is denied the same right to choose treatment for illness as the person who is physically ill. One may prefer not to undergo treatment because of the stigma still placed on mental illness. Full-time involuntary hospitalization should be ordered only as a last resort. Persons suffering from mental illness who are not alleged to have committed any crime should not be totally deprived of their liberty if there are less drastic or restrictive means for accomplishing the same basic treatment goals. To comply with constitutional guarantees of due process, equal protection of the law, and freedom from cruel and unusual punishment, legislative abridgment to fundamental personal liberties through involuntary civil commitment of the mentally ill must provide for use of the least restrictive alternatives to achieve the desired treatment.

Where an emergency exists and immediate action is required to save a patient's life or prevent permanent impairment of the client's health, and it is not possible to obtain consent of the patient or someone legally authorized to give consent, the procedure may be undertaken without liability for failure to procure consent. This rule applies when a condition that must be corrected immediately is discovered during an operation and consent of the client or someone authorized to give consent cannot be obtained. The privilege to proceed in emergency situations without consent is accorded because inaction at such a time may cause greater injury and be contrary to good medical practice. The court may find there is an implied consent. The medical care provider should document the facts and circumstances, including why consent could not be obtained.

Adult clients who are conscious and mentally competent have the right to refuse any medical or surgical procedure. This refusal must be honored whether it is grounded in doubt that the contemplated procedure will be successful, concern about the proper or possible results, lack of confidence in the physician or surgeon, religious belief, or mere whim. Every person has the legal right to refuse to permit a touching of his or her body; failure to respect this right may result in liability for assault and battery or for performance of a procedure without informed consent.

Nurses have two main duties with respect to a client's consent to treatment. First, nurses generally assume responsibility for completing the consent form, delivering it to the patient, explaining the medical procedures in language comprehensible to the patient, and obtaining the patient's consent. Second, after an initial consent has been procured, nurses must notify the hospital administration of any changes in a client's consent.

It is sometimes difficult to simultaneously explain a procedure clearly, to satisfy the legal requirement that the client understand, and to avoid frightening the client. Much discretion and care are required to avoid over- or underemphasis of the risks.

Thus, it is preferable that the client's consent be procured by the operating physician since the physician, who knows best what the diagnosis is and what the treatment or operative procedure involves, is best equipped to impart the necessary information for obtaining a valid consent and best able to answer the client's questions. Further, if the consent is invalid, the physician will be liable, not the nurse, even if the nurse obtained the signature on the consent form. The discussion of the client's condition and recommended treatment also provides an excellent opportunity for establishing a more desirable physician–client relationship. If the client feels that the physician cares, he or she may be less inclined to sue, even if an error is made.

Some states, such as Louisiana, have statutes that stipulate what is to be included in a consent form. Nurses qualified to obtain a patient's consent should be familiar with the law and practice in the area and be certain that the consent obtained conforms thereto. Two witnesses should usually be asked to sign the form, and, in selecting witnesses, the nurse should always select persons who can be located if a suit should be brought at a later time. Some statutes provide that consent is implied if a patient is unconscious and unable to do so. Such statutes include those for blood, urine, and breath tests when there is a suspicion that a driver was drunk. Patients may withdraw consent at any time; the withdrawal may be oral even if the original consent was in writing.

CRIMINAL LAW AND THE NURSE PRACTITIONER[44]

Drugs and Medications

All states have promulgated statutes specifying that pharmacy may be practiced only by legally licensed persons. The individual statutes also define those activities that constitute the practice of pharmacy. Although the definitions vary from state to state, certain activities are common to all of the definitions.

Essentially, the practice of pharmacy includes preparing, compounding, dispensing, and retailing drugs, medicines, prescriptions, chemicals, and poisons. These activities may be carried out only by a pharmacist with a state license or by a person exempted from the provisions of the state's pharmacy statute. A physician is such an exempted person when he or she compounds, dispenses, or administers medicines or drugs to clients during practice. A nurse is also exempt from the prohibitions of the various pharmacy statutes when administering a medicine or drug to a client on the oral or written order of a physician. Any nurse who administers a drug without order from a physician is in violation of the state's pharmacy statute.

To abide by the provisions of the state pharmacy acts, nurses should understand what specific activities constitute the compounding, dispensing, and retailing of pharmaceutical items.

Compounding is the combining and mixing of drugs, chemicals, or poisons. For example, a pharmacist compounds a drug by filling a physician's prescription, since this entails preparing and mixing the prescribed articles.

Dispensing is defined as delivering, distributing, disposing, or giving away a drug, medicine, prescription, chemical, or poison. Although some state statutes authorize nurses to dispense drugs in certain instances, most states do not provide such specific statutory authorization. Theoretically, nurses may not dispense drugs in states that do not provide specific authorization. However, in many hospitals it is the general practice and custom to allow nurses to enter the hospital pharmacy and obtain or remove drugs from the hospital's floor stock cabinet in order to carry out a physician's orders. Despite this generally accepted practice, the restrictions in the state pharmacy acts have been modified very little.

Retailing is simply the act of selling or trading a drug, medicine, prescription, chemical, or poison.

The articles that are compounded and dispensed by a pharmacist are drugs, medicines, prescriptions, chemicals, and poisons. The definition of *drug* in most state statutes is similar to that found in the Federal Food, Drug, and Cosmetic Act, which states that drugs are articles recognized in the official *United States Pharmacopoeia,* official *Homeopathic Pharmacopoeia of the United States,* or official *National Formulary,* or their supplements, and articles other than food intended to affect the structure or function of the body of man or other animals.

Applying this definition, courts have decided that aspirin, laxatives, vitamin and mineral capsules, honey, and whole human blood can be drugs under certain circumstances. Therefore, when handling these drugs, nurses should be aware that they cannot be dispensed, compounded, or retailed.

Violation of the pharmacy acts may be evidence of negligence, but there has been no court decision holding a nurse negligent because the action which resulted in harm was also in violation of the state pharmacy act.

Although state pharmacy acts define the minimum qualifications for dispensing drugs, nurse licensing laws may also provide standards of practice relevant to drug dispensing. For example, in Louisiana, licensed practical nurses are not permitted to give intravenous injections, because of the greater risk in giving such medications. Only graduate, professional nurses are permitted to give them.

Violation of a licensing statute can produce liability only when it can be proved that the violation was the cause of the harm. If it is foreseeable that harm may result if an unlicensed person performs acts that are restricted to licensed persons with professional training and experience, and if an unlicensed person performs such an act and in fact causes harm, liability will be imposed. However, when no harm results from the violation of a licensing statute, the appropriate state licensing board must decide whether to prosecute for its violation.

Almost all drugs handled and administered by nurses are rigidly regulated, and every nurse who is authorized to deal with these drugs must understand the manner in which they are regulated. The Federal Food, Drug and Cosmetic Act applies to the purity, labelling, potency, safety, and effectiveness of various products in varying degrees, depending on how they are classified. The Comprehensive Drug Abuse Prevention and Control Act of 1970 regulates the dispensing of controlled substances.

The term "practitioner" is defined by the statute to be a physician, dentist, veterinarian, scientific investigator, pharmacy, hospital, or other person licensed, registered, or otherwise permitted, by the United States or the jurisdiction in which the individual practices or does research, to distribute, dispense, or administer a controlled substance in the course of professional practice or research.

The term "dispense" means to deliver a controlled substance to an ultimate user or research subject by, or pursuant to the lawful order of, a practitioner, including the prescribing and administering of a controlled substance.

The term "administer" refers to the direct application of a controlled substance to the body of a patient or research subject by—

a. A practitioner (or in his or her absence, by an authorized agent), or
b. The patient or research subject at the direction and in the presence of the practitioner, whether such application be by injection, inhalation, ingestion, or any other means.

These sections of the Controlled Substances Act indicate that a nurse is prohibited from prescribing controlled substances. However, a nurse is authorized to administer a controlled substance at the direction of a practitioner. Thus, a nurse may follow a physician's oral and written orders to administer or dispense a prescribed quantity of a drug at a specified time to the proper patient. The physician need not be present at the time the controlled substance is dispensed or administered by the nurse in accordance with the physician's orders.

LEGAL REPORTING OBLIGATIONS[45]

Statutes require that there be a report made by medical care providers of certain facts and conditions. These include ophthalmia neonatorum, phenylketonuria in newborns, communicable diseases, gunshot wounds, battered wives, and abused children. The latter two have received particular emphasis and constitute grave medical, social, and legal problems of our society. Criminal penalties, as well as civil liability, have been imposed in some states for failure to report.

GOOD SAMARITAN LAWS

Most states have enacted good samaritan laws that relieve physicians, nurses, and in some instances laypersons from liability in certain emergency situations. Good samaritan legislation encourages health professionals to render assistance at the scene of an emergency. By offering immunity, the laws attempt to overcome the widespread notion that physicians, nurses, and others who render assistance in emergencies are likely to be held liable for negligence. Some states have recently enacted good samaritan laws applicable to emergency medical care providers such as emergency medical technicians, medics, and ambulance attendants.

LICENSING LAWS AND SCOPE OF PRACTICE[46]

The practice of medicine, nursing, and practical nursing are all regulated by state statutes. Failure to observe a license to practice does not in itself imply a presumption or inference of negligence, nor does it constitute negligence per se.

A plaintiff must allege and prove injury resulting from the unlicensed practitioner's negligence or lack of skill. The standard of care and skill against which the actions of the unlicensed nurse are measured is the one prevailing among properly licensed nurses, physicians, or practical nurses.

A client may delay proper treatment and be hampered by the delay because of reliance on diagnosis and treatment of an unlicensed person. To establish proximate cause for the injury, it may be sufficient to show that the delay of proper treatment resulted in the injury, even though the unlicensed nurse's, physician's, or practical nurse's treatment itself may not have caused the injury.

Whether risks of suits for malpractice will be increased or decreased by the use of nurse practitioners and physician assistants remains to be determined. It is possible that malpractice suits will decrease because physicians' time will be conserved to permit them to exercise greater care in their functions. Greater patient satisfaction may result because of the involvement of nurse practitioners and physician assistants and because physicians will have more time to involve themselves with their patients.

There are significant differences among the states in education, regulation, and reimbursement of nurse practitioners and physician assistants. The increase in the number of nurse practitioners and physician assistants has brought to light the need for legislation and regulation. Proliferation of training programs, availability of professional opportunities, and method of third-party reimbursement will determine the future for nurse practitioners. As opportunities expand and roles change, so will legislation and regulation.

The degree of physician supervision required varies among the states and is not clearly defined. Nurse practitioners and physician assistants practicing in rural areas are not required to have as great a degree of supervision as those employed by hospitals or physicians. The report of the study of the United States Department of Health, Education, and Welfare (HEW), *Review and Analysis of State Legislation and Reimbursement Practices of Physician's Assistants and Nurse Practitioners,* published in January 1978, reflects a lack of clarity in the legislation of many states, a lack of uniformity among the states, and a lack of conceptual ties between interstate regulations and reimbursement practices. The study points out the necessity of further defining the guidelines for practices of nurse practitioners and physician assistants and for more extensive investigation of practice patterns such as physician supervision, drug dispensing, regulation of practices, and education and reimbursement.

Among the primary causes of the medical malpractice crisis are poor quality and high cost of medical care and a poor personal relationship between client and physician. Use of nurse practitioners and physician assistants may reduce medical malpractice actions by obtaining a greater degree of patient satisfaction. Performance of tasks formerly limited to physicians should provide the physician with extra time, enabling him or her to function more competently by taking advantage of continuing education and by having more time to devote to the management of the client's care and treatment. More personalized attention can be devoted by the physician as well as the nurse practitioner and physician assistant. This should establish a better personal relationship with the client. If a client likes the health care provider, the patient may hesitate to sue. As a result of more time spent with the clients than the physician could devote, the nurse practitioner may observe signs, symptoms, and problems more readily than the physician, and timely institution of proper care and treatment may reduce the probability of injury from failure to diagnose and treat. The quality of care can be improved with reduction in malpractice actions. On the other hand, if nurse practitioner and physician assistant programs do not properly prepare the students for the responsibilities placed upon them, and if physicians use them to increase their practice, then the quality of care may be poor and the medical malpractice crisis may become more severe.

Regulation of education and licensing to assure competence is essential. The degree of physician supervision needed will depend on the education and competency of nurse practitioners and physician assistants. When the health care provider is competent and the quality of care is high, the likelihood of injury due to negligence is less and it follows that the number of suits for malpractice will decrease.

The medical profession may be reluctant to relinquish control over what has traditionally been considered the practice of medicine. Certainly, consumer safety must be considered in determining the extent of permitted performance, particularly unsupervised care by nurse practitioners and physician assistants. Perhaps a guide for this determination will come from observation of care rendered in rural areas under less supervision and from comparison of performance of nurse practitioners and physician assistants with that of physicians.

The legal standards for determining liability of nurse practitioners and physician assistants will be the same as previously discussed. The community standard and what the reasonable nurse practitioner and physician assistant should do under the circumstances will be determined by the jury based on evidence of what the nursing and medical professions consider proper practice for these new health professionals and on legislation regulating their practice. If they practice under supervision and control of their employers—a hospital and/or a physician—then the employer will be liable under the doctrine of *respondeat superior.* Under the good samaritan acts of some states, immunity from liability has been granted to paramedics in emergency situations, unless they have been grossly negligent.

Patterns of regulation and reimbursement by third parties to nurse practitioners and physician assistants will probably continue to change, as will the extent of their practice. With increase in responsibilities there is a greater probability of being sued. The future of these new midlevel professionals depends on educational and employment opportunities and third-party reimbursement. The need for future analyses and an update on a regular basis has been recommended to HEW.

Those practicing without licenses may be criminally prosecuted for doing so. Persons holding themselves out as nurse practitioners should consult with the medical and nursing boards within their respective states and review the licensing statutes to be certain that the medical care they render conforms with what is permitted under the laws of the particular states in which they practice. Otherwise, nurse practitioners could subject themselves to criminal prosecution as well as civil liability.

NOTES

1. *Self-pronouncing Law Dictionary* (Lawyers Cooperative Publishing Company 1948), p. 160.

2. J. Fleming, Jr., *Civil Procedure,* ed. 1 (1965), pp. 31–45. M. W. Cazalas, "Legalities and Nursing," *Association of Operating Room Nurses Journal* 13, no. 5 (1971): 79–80.

3. M. W. Cazalas, "Legalities and Nursing," *Association of Operating Room Nurses Journal* 13, no. 5 (1978): 80.

4. Ibid.

5. Ibid.

6. Ibid.

7. Ibid.

8. Ibid.

9. A. Averbach, *Handling Accident Cases,* Vol. 3A, (Lawyers Cooperative Publishing Company, 1970), Section 79, p. 417.

10. Ibid., pp. 419–420.

11. Ibid., pp. 420–422.

12. R. J. Hunter, *Federal Trial Handbook* (Lawyers Cooperative Publishing Company, 1974) pp. 525–535.

13. Ibid., pp. 535, 540, 541.

14. Ibid., pp. 530–533, 540–541.

15. M. W. Cazalas, *Nursing and the Law,* 3d ed. (Germantown, Maryland: Aspen Systems Corporation, 1978), pp. 51–58.

16. Ibid.

17. Ibid.

18. Hunter, pp. 503–504.

19. Ibid.

20. *Nursing and the Law.*

21. Hunter, pp. 410–413.

22. *Nursing and the Law.*

23. Ibid.

24. Ibid.

25. Ibid.

26. Ibid.

27. Ibid.

28. Ibid.

29. Hunter, pp. 580–581, 331–344.

30. Ibid., pp. 580–581.

31. Ibid., pp. 45–51.

32. Ibid., pp. 48–51.

33. Ibid.

34. Ibid., pp. 44–51.

35. Ibid.

36. Ibid.
37. Ibid.
38. *Nursing and the Law,* pp. 17–25.
39. Ibid., pp. 101, 103–106.
40. Averbach, pp. 111–117.
41. *Nursing and the Law,* pp. 27–30.
42. Ibid., pp. 69–75.
43. Ibid., pp. 31–49.
44. Ibid., pp. 59–67.
45. Ibid., pp. 145–152.
46. Ibid., pp. 79–92.

Chapter 13

Quality Assurance

ACCOUNTABILITY

Nursing and the law presently interface to a greater extent than ever before. The public is demanding more health care accountability, and nursing is increasingly striving to demonstrate its provision of accountability. Health care literature is full of articles and information on the topic, resulting in a public and professional concern with accountability.

Considerable emphasis is placed on the individual nurse's responsibility, demanding informed and mature judgments in all nursing roles. Individual responsibility is the key to contemporary nursing. It is the major contributing factor to nursing's growth to its present level of sophistication.

Nurses in any setting are responsible and accountable for their acts. Whether a traditional hospital setting or a new private nursing practice, the same level of responsibility is expected. Decision making can have the same high quality in private practice as in a hospital setting, because nurses in each setting can collaborate with colleagues and others regarding their clients' care. The nurse in private practice is not isolated, alone, and independent. Collaboration is an essential, expected, and required part of quality nursing practice.

Nurses should grasp opportunities to organize care in a fashion that will minimize the client's health care fragmentation. Nurses must constantly recognize their obligation to their clients and aim for the best health care regimen for the client. These responsibilities are not limited to nurses in private practice; they apply to nurses in all situations.

All nurses must have a knowledge of the governmental legislation that affects the health care they provide. While all nurses make independent decisions about clients and provide nursing care based on their independent decisions at times, nurses in any setting could not be considered totally independent nurse practitioners. Their independent decisions are formulated from collaboration with others, although actually performing the care may be done solely by the nurse.

Jordan says that nursing has already advanced in accountability. Nursing's defined and implemented standards for entry into the profession demonstrate this fact. A national examining system for public safety has been established. Each state has defined nursing practice, and laws regulate nursing practice accordingly. These laws impose penalties on violators. License revocation is a penalty for incompetence and gross negligence. Nurses are held accountable for ethical and legal acts.

Nursing is moving toward a shared governance and parity with physicians. This trend can only create optimum care for clients. Collaboration among health care disciplines is becoming increasingly important.[1]

Demonstrating Accountability

Nurses in private practice can demonstrate accountability to their clients and the public in various ways. They can hang their framed nursing license where it is visible to others. They can also display nursing diplomas, degrees, awards, or special honors as well as letters endorsing or supporting the private practice.

These professional techniques are widely accepted by the public and constitute additional proof of your capabilities and professionalism. Your professional care to your clients is the most important way to demonstrate accountability.

Negligence and Liability

All nurses, as licensed individuals, are responsible to their clients and their families for maintaining standards of practice. Malpractice is the term for negligence or carelessness on the part of professionals. The law has developed a measuring tool to determine careless acts. This tool is the standard of care, which is determined by deciding what a reasonable, prudent person would do under similar conditions. A judge or jury makes the determination. Negligence can constitute either acts of commission or omission, Cazalas explains.[2]

Greighton summarizes that nurses who, in any manner, aid in the injury to clients can be sued for those injuries by the client regardless of who employs the nurse or whether the nursing care was given for pay or gratuitously. Whether the nurse is an independent contractor or an employee of an institution is important to determine the liability of other persons.[3]

Consumerism

Arndt and Huckabay report that the American Nurses Association and the National League for Nursing, along with the community, set a goal concerning a client's right to expect high-quality care and personal nursing service. These expectations should become reality as nursing becomes more accountable through evaluating client care.[4]

Rothman and Rothman explain that John F. Kennedy set forth a Consumer Bill of Rights. This bill included:

- the right to safety
- the right to be informed
- the right to choose
- the right to be heard

Health care consumers are increasingly more cognizant of their rights. They expect these rights in greater frequency and demand them when they are not provided. Within the last ten years interest has increased in consumerism as it relates to the health care disciplines.[5]

Nurses today are involved with a heightened societal awareness of the needs and rights of consumers to achieve optimum health care. Professionals acquire and maintain authority over their practices by demonstrating that they are publicly answerable to their clients.

Safety in Role Transfer

The responsibility and role transfer from physician to nurse has been very slow. Traditional institutions of nursing employment are reluctant to allow responsibility or role transfer to competent, willing nurses. This reluctance may be due to pressure from medical associations, lack of nursing role clarity, or administrators' threatened feelings.

Often physicians are unwilling to transfer roles or responsibility to nurses because they feel the nurses are incompetent. Physicians themselves may not clearly understand their role.

Nurses themselves are reluctant to take on more responsibility because of fears or uncertainty. Prudent nurses will not accept additional roles if the setting they are practicing in does not have enough staff to allow for it, or if they know they are not capable of it.

Current roles can be role retreats or escapes when new roles are offered. In the proper setting, it would be professional and proper for the practicing nurse to accept more responsibilities and more sophisticated roles. Nurses who collaborate professionally with physicians may find physicians willing to transfer more activities and roles.

To minimize nurses' legal and moral trepidation, they should remember not to take on roles they cannot perform or that are esoterically reserved for the physician. Collaboration with colleagues will aid in determining these roles. Explain your point of view for not performing the care to the physician; request that the physician teach the procedure to you, so that you could perform the care. If you then feel competent, accept the role transfer.

Be certain to incorporate the safety mechanisms explained in Chapter 2. Implementation of the nursing process throughout all clients' care will also help to ensure safety, quality assurance, and quality control. Many other evaluative methods exist for quality assurance; some of them follow.

Peer Review

Nursing can benefit by self-policing or peer review. Peer review means peer control. Thus, nurses would evaluate the nursing care provided by other nurses. Nurses need to be magnanimous and methodical enough to accept this new policy.

Guidelines for peer review are needed from governing authorities and associations. You may want to confer with or hire colleagues to review your private practice and your nursing care. These evaluations could be ongoing or sporadic. Constructive criticism may prove valuable if it comes from an outside and objective point of view. It is wise to listen to suggestions and implement appropriate ones.

Peer review is popular; it is only beginning to come into its own as a substantial method for controlling the quality of nursing practice. Peer review boards and centers are needed on a large scale; they should be utilized liberally in examinations of private nurse practitioners.

Far too often nurses encounter hostility from their peers when they raise legitimate questions about the quality of client care. There is no need for this hostility. Nursing will become more viable once peer review is implemented in a well-planned and practical fashion. The danger from overzealous nurses asking questions is less than the danger from a nursing profession unwilling to exercise its responsibility and authority to ensure professionalism.

A barrier to accountability involves implementation—a guarantee of honest and meaningful peer review. Peer review is becoming commonplace to health care; however, more development is needed to ensure accountability. Peer review can focus on the client or on the professional, McClure explains. Peer review that focuses on the client is the most widely used. Usually, health care agencies have committees that carry out peer review.[6]

Honesty is extremely important. It is easy to be misled by feelings that nurses should practice conspiracy of silence as other professionals may. It may be best to confer with nurses you think are practicing improperly before making any official reports on what you feel may be misconduct. Conferring with them may enlighten you to the fact that they were practicing properly. And, if they were practicing improperly, usually a word to the wise is sufficient. Your re-educating could be all the peer review that is needed. When this fails, officiating a report may be necessary.

Horsley says that nurses should not be led astray by the idea that nurses should not report one another. Juries and judges view it as a cover-up. Reporting misconduct may save lives and prevent disabilities.

Nurses who do not report colleagues' wrong doings, physicians included, are liable of malpractice. Plaintiff's attorneys are aware of the nurse's responsibility to report misconduct or malpractice by other health care personnel.[7]

The United States Congress recently passed legislation (P.L. 92-603) calling for Professional Service Review Organizations (PSROs), says Ramphal. This law is evidence of public pressure for meaningful regulation of costs and quality of health care. PSRO is a governmental attempt to include consumer participation in the planning of health services. Already nursing has responded to public demands for mandatory continuing education for licensure, consumer participation in planning of health services, and consumer participation in state licensing boards.

Governmental regulation of costs and quality may produce constraints detrimental to the public. Nursing needs to participate in peer review to ensure the quality of practice, thus regulating decision making of health services and standards.[8]

Nursing Audit

The purpose of a nursing audit is to find methods of improving client care. Nurses are excellent sources of information about client care. Other nurses can audit your clients' records, your private practice, and you. They have much to offer towards improvement of care.

Records are frequently examined in an audit. Be certain to keep good ones. The proper mechanics must be adhered to in clients' charts. Audits are for the clients' and the nurses' concern. A well-executed audit can keep clients from harm and reduce the possibility of negligent care, malpractice suits, or legal investigations.

Whoever performs the nursing audit must define the nursing practice criteria. Then the nursing care that was offered should be compared systematically with the criteria. From this comparison, a decision can be made whether an acceptable level of nursing practice was provided. Documentation of nursing care is definitely needed so that nurses can prove the quality of care they offered.

The Joint Commission on Accreditation of Hospitals (JCAH) requires nursing audits. It also requires follow-up with another audit to determine whether corrective action was taken and whether it was effective. Perhaps JCAH could become involved with auditing private nursing practices.

Ganong and Ganong point out that JCAH is a hospital governing body with ultimate responsibility for the quality of care. JCAH delegates the evaluation process of client care to administration. The nursing and medical staff can use any method they choose to perform the audit; however, the audit must include:

1. standards and criteria of care sought
2. measurement of care provided versus the criteria and standards
3. evaluation of this measurement
4. deficiency corrective action
5. follow-up and re-evaluation
6. reports to nursing and medical services and to administration[9]

Ethics

One way professionals can act collectively to ensure safe and quality practice is to follow ethical codes. These codes should define professional responsibility and the professional-client relationship.

Levine says that nursing relationships begin with ethical responsibility. While clients may always be able to choose a physician, they cannot always choose their nurse. The client is dependent on the nurse and must assume the nursing care received is safe and effective and that the nurse is ethically and morally responsible and accountable.[10]

Nursing is a profession in transition. In this transition, constant awareness of your professional behavior will pay off in a moral, ethical, and legal practice. Contacting your regulatory or governing agency for a code of ethics is advised. The American Nurses Association has a booklet entitled *Code for Nurses with Interpretative Statements;* you may wish to write for it.

Table 13-1 lists ethics that apply to the overall practice of nursing, but should definitely be applied to private nursing practice.

Investigations

If your practice is investigated, you should feel confident, provided you have practiced morally, ethically, and legally. In fact, an investigation could prove beneficial to you, nursing, the investigators, and the investigating agency as all can learn and benefit by it.

Table 13-1 Ethics for Nurses in Private Practice

1. Provide your clients with respectful care.
2. Do not discriminate among your clients for any reason.
3. Maintain confidentiality.
4. Become involved with continuing education for the benefit of you and your clients.
5. Be responsible for your actions.
6. Use judgment when accepting responsibility in order to practice nursing safely.
7. Be active in upgrading the nursing profession.
8. Maintain high quality nursing care.
9. Practice nursing interdependently.
10. Refrain from advertising or promotion of particular products for sale.
11. Consider your clients' emotional needs.
12. Communicate with your clients.
13. Inform the clients of the fee for the service beforehand.
14. Explain your bills to the clients and allow them to examine the bills before payment.
15. Allow the clients time, if needed, to pay fees.
16. Keep adequate records.
17. Never falsify records.
18. Obtain physicians' orders as needed.
19. Collaborate with colleagues often.
20. Wear a badge indicating your name and professional status.
21. Practice within the realm of nursing.
22. Never give or take a fee or other consideration from a third party for the referral of a client.
23. Do not allow another person to share in the fees for your nursing service unless the other person is a partner, employee, or someone professionally and directly associated with you.
24. When delegating responsibility, be certain that person is legally trained for the responsibility, licensed, and capable of performing the task.
25. Refrain from making claims of professional superiority.
26. Never abandon or neglect your client under care or in need of immediate care, without making reasonable arrangements for the continuation of care.
27. Refrain from immoral conduct with your clients.

An investigation can be intimidating and frightening, as was the one in the second year my practice was in operation. Two inspectors from the Professional Conduct Bureau visited the private practice. The Professional Conduct Bureau is a division of the State Education Department that polices professionals licensed by that department.

The inspectors entered the practice asking to see me. I was in Wisconsin at a research meeting regarding role changes in nursing. Another nurse, who was in charge for the time, responded to the investigators. They asked only two questions. The first was, "What would you do if I asked you to take my blood pressure?" The second was, "Would you give me the results if you took it?" The answers were that nurses at the private practice would not only take the blood pressure reading but would give the client the results. At this point, the inspectors identified themselves, explaining where they were from and that the answers to the questions created a serious problem for the private practice and its nurses. They said we would hear from them, and then they left. They also explained before leaving that taking blood pressures without physicians' orders was practicing medicine and giving the clients the results was making a diagnosis.

I was phoned in Wisconsin and returned the next day. I visited the executive director of the local district's state nursing association. The executive director provided a great deal of emotional support and aided in preparing a defense for the investigation. The executive director knew the inspectors because they collaborated almost daily regarding quality control of nursing.

Having kept the governing bodies and associations informed of the intentions of the private practice proved to be a significant aid, as the local executive director knew exactly what the private practice was all about, even though contact at the local level had never been made before. It was as if the local association had already done a peer review on the private practice. The executive director was in favor of this concept of nursing practice and supported the private practice in explaining it to the investigators.

Exhibits in triplicate of actual cases were prepared for the investigators. Several letters were sent, and many phone calls and visits were made to the executive director's office and the investigators' office. In about one month the investigation was completed. The state nurses association participated in supporting the private practice throughout the investigation.

We never learned how the investigation was triggered. The investigators were not nurses; they had an antiquated concept of what nurses were doing. The investigation proved beneficial to the private practice and its staff, because they were able to demonstrate their professionalism. They were not charged with any wrongdoing. It was determined that nurses are allowed to take blood pressures without physicians' orders and that nurses may give clients the results. It was further determined that the private practice was a professional, accepted mode of practicing nursing.

The nursing profession benefited as this investigation paved the way for other nurses in any setting to take blood pressure readings in similar fashion or to enter private practice. The investigators benefited in that they were tactfully educated to the current roles in nursing; this also benefited nursing.

Shortly after the investigation, my friend who covered the practice when the investigation began and I were invited by the local executive director to present the concept of private practice to a local meeting of members. The presentation went well. It was explained how well the state and especially the local association helped to defend nursing's role as private nurse practitioners. The members were elated.

SUMMARY

The highest level of risk taking is accountability, which nurtures the public as well as the nursing profession. Montange explains that regarding professions, the most common way to protect consumers is to restrict admission to the educational institutions needed to become a professional. Other protection devices include licensing, licensing exams, self-regulation, malpractice litigation, and governmental regulation. Licensing and restrictive admissions increase the possibility that professions will be made up of members who display an ability to integrate a complex body of learning. However, controls must keep pace with changes in ever-developing professions.[11]

Recordkeeping and client data should always be kept confidential. Confidentiality should be maintained throughout audits, reviews, and investigations.

Nurses should not be resentful when being reviewed or investigated. The investigation can aid you, nursing, and clients. If you are practicing illegally, unethically, or immorally, the review, audit, or investigation may aid nursing and clients.

NOTES

1. Clifford A. Jordan, R.N., B.S., Ed.D., "Accountability for Nursing Practice," *AORN Journal* 27, no. 6 (May 1978): 1078.

2. Mary W. Cazalas, R.N., J.D., *Nursing and the Law* (Germantown, Maryland: Aspen Systems Corporation, 1978), p. 1218.

3. Helen Greighton, R.N., B.S.N., A.B., A.M., M.S.N., J.D., *Law Every Nurse Should Know* (Philadelphia: W.B. Saunders Company, 1975), p. 79.

4. Clara Arndt, R.N., M.S., and Loucine M. Daderian Huckabay, R.N., B.S., M.S., Ph.D., *Nursing Administration* (St. Louis: The C.V. Mosby Company, 1975), p. 72.

5. Daniel Rothman, A.J.D., and Lloyd Nancy Rothman, R.N., B.S.N., M.Ed., *The Professional Nurse and the Law* (Boston: Little, Brown and Company, 1977), pp. 83–4.

6. Margaret L. McClure, R.N., Ed.D., "The Long Road to Accountability," *Nursing Outlook* 26, no. 1 (January 1978): 49–50.

7. Jack E. Horsley, K.D., "When to 'Tattle' on Physician Misconduct," *RN* 41, no. 12 (December 1978): 24.

8. Marjorie Ramphal, B.S., M.S., Ed.D., "Peer Review," *American Journal of Nursing* 74, no. 1 (January 1974): 63, 64, 66, 67.

9. Joan M. Ganong, R.N., M.S., and Warren L. Ganong, C.M.C., *Nursing Management* (Germantown, Maryland: Aspen Systems Corporation, 1976), p. 139.

10. Myra E. Levine, "Nursing Ethics and the Ethical Nurse," *American Journal of Nursing* 77, no. 5 (May 1977): 846.

11. Charles H. Montange, J.D., "Consumer Protection and Professional Services," *The Journal of Legal Medicine* 4, no. 5 (May 1976): 24.

Part IV

The Future of Private Practice

Chapter 14

Legislation—The Key to Removing Barriers

HEALTH INSURANCE MYSTIQUE

Health insurance programs and bills seem almost impossible to decipher and understand; their costs are almost as impossible to afford. Deductibles and coverage vary with each policy whether the carriers are public or private. Also, coverage by one carrier can vary from state to state.

Trying to understand insurance is extremely difficult, especially for the elderly. In spite of all the fancy wording (coverage, noncoverage, costs to consumers, and claims of extended coverage), no insurance provides the consumer with the freedom to choose nursing care on a fee-for-service basis.

Ubell says that there are over 1,500 health insurance carriers in America. They offer basic to broad coverage. Regardless of how expensive your insurance coverage is, you can still be vulnerable to devastating medical expenses. The consumer should beware as the responsibility to see that coverage is adequate is the consumer's alone.[1]

Health care is a major national industry. Health care costs and fiscal management have become major concerns almost simultaneously. Nursing should become involved politically with health care and health care costs and insurance; nurses should demand to be reimbursed on a fee-for-service basis.

The idea of reimbursement for nursing care on a fee-for-service basis will force nurses to look at issues they formerly avoided. Nurses have been providing care at lower costs than physicians. They also provide care in areas where and when physicians are not available.

Third-party payment or fee-for-service reimbursement for nurses practicing privately is long overdue. Practicing privately means entrepreneurially independent but not independent nursing; collaboration with others regarding client care is a basic part of the job. Reimbursement directly to nurses along with removal of the requirement of physically immediate medical supervision would encourage qualified nurses to provide greater care in unserved areas.

The answers to this problem lie in legislation. Nurses should not only have parity with physicians in regard to overlapping of roles and their responsibilities but should have pay parity that is reflected in third-party reimbursement.

Governmental oppression of nurses has hindered American public health care for too long. This oppression has been concealed in an intricate web of quasi-legal rules and regulations. Nurses today need a thorough understanding of the legal system to enable them to respond to the political process of litigation. Thus, the American Nurses Association has a lobby to decipher these rules and regulations and to help incorporate nurses into them more fully for the benefit of the public and nursing.

National Health Insurance

Nurses may achieve recognition from health insurance plans in a new forthcoming plan: National Health Insurance (NHI). Since this plan is in its developmental stages, nursing has the opportunity to lobby to ensure the inclusion of nurses on a fee-for-service basis in NHI. Whether pay parity occurs at the onset is secondary to being included. Pay parity could come after nurses demonstrate their capabilities with fee-for-service inclusion in NHI and the benefits afforded to all by their inclusion.

According to Wehr, President Carter says that any national health insurance should assure that all Americans have comprehensive health care coverage along with quality of care. They should have the freedom to choose their physicians, hospitals, and health delivery systems. The plan should be noninflationary. The president has given a directive to Secretary of Health, Education and Welfare, Joseph A. Califano, Jr., to draft a health plan to be submitted to Congress in 1979.[2]

Existing health care systems and plans have defects that should be corrected. At least 20 million Americans do not have health care, and 65 million face possible bankruptcy because their insurance does not provide enough coverage. Health care resources are poorly distributed; thus rural and inner city areas experience gaps in services. America's health care personnel are among the finest; their strengths should be drawn upon in more useful ways.

NHI should assure that all Americans have ample coverage and the freedom to choose a provider. It should provide payment to increase the availability of ambulatory and preventive care. The inclusion of nurses to greater extents will do just that.

Plans for NHI seem to include everything and everyone related to health care delivery except nurses. This "fresh new plan" should have included nurses on a fee-for-service basis at its inception. Why hasn't nursing confronted the lack of recognition in this plan?

Mauksch says that nursing's ability to care for the public to its fullest potential has been limited by lack of reimbursement for nursing services. The fact that people cannot acquire nursing services without physician approval has also hurt nursing's potential. NHI would enable nurses to care for more people, more appropriately, if nurses were reimbursed on a fee-for-service basis.[3]

Vogl says that Cohen, the father of Medicare, feels nurses must be included in NHI on a fee-for-service basis. Nurses must be put into a position that is compatible with their professional ideals. Also, they must be reimbursed in a way that is acceptable to them.

The goal of NHI is not necessarily cost containment but rather distribution of costs in a more rational manner. Ways to make more intelligent use of health personnel must be found. The number of neighborhood health centers has to expand, particularly in the inner cities. Nurses deserve a larger role in NHI.[4] Legislators should create and pass bills to include nurses in fee schedules of public and private insurance plans on a fee-for-service basis. The very legislators who oppose these bills may very well eventually suffer from the lack of nursing care they perpetuated.

Wehr explains that the Senate decided to invest a half-billion dollars in nurses' education during 1979 and 1980. This action rejected President Carter's claim that there were enough nurses already. The Senate, on June 7, 1978, passed a reauthorization bill (S. 2416) by voice vote; it was sponsored by Jacob Javits, R-N.Y. The House passed H.R. 12303, a similar bill. Each continues funds at current levels to 1980 for construction or renovation of schools of nursing, capitation grants, and special projects for advanced training and special purposes.

President Carter proposed only to maintain the special projects funds at half the current level and nurse practitioner training funds for a total of $20 million. President Carter feels there are enough nurses and that this funding can be cut. Jacob K. Javits is not convinced there are enough nurses now or in the future.

The May 15 report (S. Rept. 95-859) on the bill by the Senate Human Resources Committee explained that hospitals were complaining of acute nursing shortages, especially in inner city and rural areas. This committee argued that these cuts in financial support would cripple nursing education and that future health policies would create more demands for nurses. The House Commerce Committee argued in its report (H. Rept. 95-1189) that NHI would affect the types and numbers of nurses needed.[5]

President Carter refused to sign these two-year reauthorization bills for nurses' education. Donsky says that nursing leaders were angered and felt that this was discriminatory. Barbara Nichols, President of the American Nurses Association, assumes that this veto had a lot to do with the fact that nursing is predominantly composed of female members.

President Carter, on November 11, 1978, announced that he would not sign S. 2416 because of its inflationary air, and that 20 years of federal aid had ended nursing shortages. Carter asked Congress to continue the special projects and nurse practitioner funds. Congress has continued a broad range of grants through 1980.

Congressional sources predicted that in 1979 funds would be added to other health legislation and suggested that Carter would be unable to kill the nursing programs. In 1975 Ford's veto had been overridden, because it is difficult to vote against nurses. There are many nurses in every district; they are effective and confront legislators with arguments of discrimination.[6]

Nurses should feel pleased that their government is expending a great deal of time and energy as well as funds to educate them; to support educational facilities; and to provide for special projects, including the education of nurse practitioners. The public, too, should be pleased. However, nurses and the public should be distressed that their government is not enabling these nurses to be available to the public. The same government that provides the nurses also inhibits the public's direct access to nursing care. Nurses are made unavailable to the public in the Medicare, Medicaid, NHI, and private insurance plans.

Medicare

Medicare is government-sponsored health insurance for people over 65 years of age. It is paid monthly through Social Security taxes on employees and employers. It currently pays for a large part of hospital bills, some physicians' bills, some medical supplies, and maybe for renal care provided by renal nurse specialists.

Recently H.R. 8423 (P.L. 95-292) was signed into law, representing a significant change in the Medicare coverage requirements. One of the main stipulations related to private nurse practitioners is that Medicare will now pay for all supplies used in home care and for periodic monitoring and maintenance visits from dialysis personnel. In this way, hopefully, private nurse practitioners who specialize in renal dialysis can be reimbursed for treating these types of clients at home.

The problem remains that Medicare personnel will either be unfamiliar with this change in the law and refuse to reimburse for this nursing care or that nurses would have to be employed by a home health agency. The requirement of having reimbursement only for home health agency employees is discriminatory in reference to nurses. Physicians receive Medicare reimbursement and are not required to be home health agencies. Why should that stipulation be required of professional, accountable nurses? Hopefully, Medicare will reimburse private nurse practitioners specializing in renal diseases for treating clients at home.

It is surprising that ranking health care professionals have not yet fully realized the capabilities and contributions of nurses. The nursing profession is responsible for continuing to demonstrate their abilities to win universal acceptance of nurses' skills. Such persistence to achieve this recognition is not new to nursing, Skipper said.[7]

The tragedy that results from nurses' exclusion from fee-for-service is felt by the public. They are forced to enter hospitals, visit physicians and emergency departments, and enter other institutions when they shouldn't have to. Their insurance plans foster only these types of care. Overcrowding, increased taxes to support Medicare payments, loneliness, and hardship to the client and client's family result. The culprit is not only Medicare but also any health insurance plan that refuses to include nurses in fee-for-service reimbursement.

The problem with Medicare is that too many conditions must be met for coverage: physician determination that services (part-time nursing) are needed and a physician plan for home care 14 days after discharge from the qualifying facility. Other requirements are proven need to be confined to your home and provision of care by a home health agency that participates with Medicare. The client must have been in a qualifying hospital for at least three days in a row, and the home care must be for further treatment of a condition that was treated in the hospital or the skilled nursing facility.

A home health agency is a public or private agency that provides specialized and skilled nursing services or other therapeutic services such as physical therapy in the home. The home health agency is considered a supplier, once its application is approved by Medicare. The supplier receives a supply code number, often called a vendor number. This code number is inserted on the request for Medicare payment filed by the supplier seeking Medicare reimbursement. Physicians do not have to make an application to receive a supplier code number.

Nurses should receive supplier code numbers for third-party payment automatically, since they are professionals who supply skilled nursing services. If supplier code numbers were not granted automatically, nursing associations could determine which nurses should receive them. Perhaps at least one year of experience and a bachelor's degree with demonstrated abilities to practice nursing in an honest and sophisticated manner could be prerequisites. Credentials reviews and professional references could aid in this determination. Whatever mechanism is employed, a majority of nurses should be found credible enough to receive Medicare recognition. Restricting qualification to a minority of nurses defeats its purpose. However, some peer review may be used to demonstrate greater professionalism than in other health disciplines. Other disciplines restrict examinations only after an unjust incident, such as abuse of the payment system. Nursing could set up credentials review quickly, thus creating peer review boards throughout America to facilitate public service. Credentials reviews can be done quickly and cheaply; they already have credibility throughout the professions—nursing included. Reviews would not be limited to Medicare but be applicable to all types of health insurance reimbursement plans, for nurses to receive fee-for-service, third-party payment.

Medicare has many benefits, but it limits the public's use of the nursing profession. The Medicaid program has wide variations from state to state regarding what benefits are available or who can make claims to them. Medicaid limits nursing accessibility to the public as Medicare does. Medicaid needs similar reform.

President Carter called for comprehensive health insurance in his 1976 platform. Since then there have been many economic problems holding it back. Nurse inclusion may help iron out these economic problems since nurses, by caring for clients at home, could reduce the cash outlay for institutional care.

Care from the Home

Home care means keeping clients out of institutions when they can receive adequate care at home. At home means from the home; patients are not necessarily bedridden or homebound. Nurse practitioners must recognize the need for institutionalization as clients' status or conditions change. Nurses may collaborate with the physician to have the client admitted to an appropriate facility when required.

Government bureaucracy is designed to protect and favor the conservative rather than the innovative. Government seems to cling to yesterday. Nurses should resist this tendency to conservatism and protect the freedom of innovation for the betterment of health care.

Birenbaum points out that there is much concern over the high cost of hospital care to consumers and third-party payers such as Blue Cross, Blue Shield, Medicare, and Medicaid. This concern leads to more extensive use of home care services. Home care costs about 25% of hospital care, since many custodial and health care tasks are carried out by the members of the household. Reducing hospitalization would reduce the total health care bill in America considerably. The development of organized care from the home depends on the health care system and its willingness to reach out.[8]

The current system of financing health services in America is disturbing. Its history reveals persistent concern with issues of equal access and equitable costs. It fails to distinguish between medical care and health care, and it is dominated by insurance plans that favor physicians, hospitals, and insurance companies themselves. Extensive waste, abuse, and corruption have occurred. The most tragic of all is the almost complete lack of recognition by the public, health care providers, and even nurses that nursing is a valuable commodity that should be afforded insurance reimbursement, says Welch.[9]

Donovan explains that if government is truly concerned about inflation, it will see caring for clients from the home as a solution to containing costs. Health insurance premiums could be held down if nurses provided more care from the home. Some clients simply can't receive proper care in the hospital, for example, the childhood diabetic. This child needs a natural environment for health regimen regulation. Nurses caring for this client from the home would enhance the treatment regimen.[10]

Rosenberg points out that Claude Pepper, Chairman of the House Select Committee on Aging, released a General Accounting Office report documenting the advantages of expanded home care. The report, *Home Health—The Need for a National Policy to Better Provide for the Elderly,* states that the cost of care in nursing homes exceeds the cost of care from the home until the elderly are extremely impaired.

Current Medicare home health requirements prevent the elderly and disabled from receiving services from their homes. A Health, Education and Welfare study shows that 14–25 percent of institutionalized elderly do not need institutionalized care.[11]

MAJOR NATIONAL HEALTH INSURANCE PLANS

There are four national health insurance plans currently proposed in Congress. Their proposals include many complex provisions, and each sponsor wants the recognition for initiating the final plan. These plans are described.

Kennedy-Corman-Labor Bill

This is a Health Security Act (S. 3, H.R. 21), sponsored by Senator Edward Kennedy, D-Mass., and Representative James Corman, D-Calif., supported by organized labor. This bill would provide federal health insurance comprehensively for the entire population. Financing would be from payroll taxes. This bill provides for quality control measures.

Long-Ribicoff-Talmadge-Dole Bill

This is the Catastrophic Health Insurance and Medical Assistance Reform Act (S. 3105), sponsored by Senators Russell Long, D-La., Abraham Ribicoff, D-Conn., Herman Talmadge, D-Ga., and Robert Dole, R-Kans. This offers catastrophic protection to the whole population and for the poor, to replace Medicaid. Employers would finance this. This follows the Medicare fee-for-service model of reimbursement.

Carter-Hansen-AMA Bill

This is the Comprehensive Health Care Insurance Act (H.R. 1818, S. 218), sponsored by Representative Tim Lee Carter, R-Ky., and Senator Clifford Hansen, R-Wyo., and is backed by the American Medical Association. Separate plans are established for employed and unemployed through private health insurance carriers.

Burleson-McIntyre-Insurance Industry Bill

This is the National Health Care Act (H.R. 5, S. 5), sponsored by Representative Omar Burleson, D-Tex., and Senator Thomas McIntyre, D-N.H. This is backed by the Health Insurance Association of America.

It is based on voluntary coverage through private carriers and a state plan for the indigent.

President Carter is considering these plans as well as a plan requiring everyone to purchase federal health insurance unless the employer provides equivalent private coverage. The latter plan gives the consumer a choice of public or private coverage.

It might be helpful for the American Nurses Association to get into the picture of National Health Insurance. Perhaps it could support a plan that would reimburse for nursing care on a fee-for-service basis. Or, perhaps the American Nurses Association could exert enough influence to encourage empathetical senators or representatives to draw up a completely new bill that would include nurses in the fee-for-service reimbursement mechanism. None of the proposed plans mention nursing, much less nursing care from the home or nurses receiving third-party payment. The fact that nurses are restricted from third-party payment is a barrier to progressive nursing care. Legislative changes to include nurses in third-party payment are the key to unlocking the barriers.

Programs for the Elderly

H.R. 10397 includes revisions for home health under Medicare and Medicaid. It adds $95 million to the Medicare 1979 budget and eliminates a two-year waiting period for disabled persons to qualify for its benefits. It also liberalizes coverage for services by dentists, optometrists, chiropractors, and clinical psychologists. But it does not increase nursing care benefits via a liberalized payment system for the elderly.

H.R. 13817 changes peer review processes, rules applying to nursing care beds in acute-care hospitals, and auditing procedures for Medicare and Medicaid. Both resolutions were passed in the second half of 1978 and ultimately aid the elderly a little more than before.

On July 24, 1978, the Senate passed a two-year extension of the Older Americans Act, the primary governmental assistance to the elderly. This legislation (S. 2850) allocated $1.2 billion for 1979 and over $1 billion for 1980. This money is for social services, health, and nutrition programs. The House passed H.R. 12255, a three-year extension of the Older Americans Act.

On May 15, 1978, the Senate Human Resources Committee reported on the bill (S. Rept. 95-8555). As passed by the Senate, the extended Older Americans Act provides increased funds for nutrition programs and home-delivered meals; it strengthens the role of the Administration on Aging in the Department of Health, Education and Welfare by making advocacy its first role. It also authorized construction for community multipurpose centers and many others.

All of these provisions for the elderly are needed and welcomed. Again, however, direct access to nurses is not mentioned.

H.R. 8422-P.L. 95-210, the Rural Health Clinics bill, extends Medicare and Medicaid reimbursement to nurse practitioners in rural health clinics. While this bill would aid the elderly, it restricts nurses from practicing in a more meaningful style since direct supervision by a physician is a prerequisite. The physician must be available to see every client a nurse sees and directly supervise it. Direct physician supervision is neither practical nor necessary. Private nurse practitioners practice from their practices, not from federally funded clinics. They do not need a physician on location to practice. They can collaborate with their clients' physicians as needed.

Hill-Burton Funds

The Hill-Burton Hospital Survey and Construction Act of 1946 was America's first major venture into health facilities planning. It provided grants-in-aid to states to partially finance hospital construction. The states were to formulate plans for regional organization of hospitals and related health facilities based on analysis of supply and demand of health care.

This Act, popularly known as the Hill-Burton Act, stipulates that any hospital receiving funds from this program must make a reasonable number of services available to indigent clients. The Act allows for federal assistance to construct public and nonprofit hospitals and health centers.

Perhaps some of the Hill-Burton Act funds could be effectively utilized by state or local nursing associations or the American Nurses Association to construct and manage nonprofit public nursing care centers, managed strictly by nurses. These centers could provide quality, varied, nursing care to clients from the home, utilizing the clients' physicians. Thus, a physician would not be needed on the premises of the nursing service center. These nursing service centers could be established throughout America; the nurses could bill on a fee-for-service basis, to further finance the center. It is possible that Hill-Burton funds would become liberalized enough to finance beginning private nurse practitioners. These funds could be made available in the form of loans or matching funds.

With or without Hill-Burton funds, nurses may wish to create Nursing Maintenance Organizations. These organizations could be profit or nonprofit, and clients could prepay, pay monthly, or pay per service. Creativity is called for in establishing greater nursing accessibility.

Acts and Bills

Senate Bill S. 104, January 15, 1975, was a bill to amend the Social Security Act to include nurses in Medicare and Medicaid. The bill was prepared by Senator Javits and associates and introduced by Senator Inouye. It would have reimbursed nurses on a fee-for-service basis. There has been little action on this bill; it can be assumed dead.

H.R. 1943, January 23, 1975, was also intended to amend the Social Security Act to include nurses in Medicare and Medicaid. Mr. Matsunaga introduced the bill and it was referred to the Committee on Ways and Means. Little action has been taken on this bill. It also would have reimbursed nurses on a fee-for-service basis.

In the New York State Assembly, bill number 5956, March 4, 1975, introduced by Mr. Blumenthal and sponsored by Mr. Silverman, Miss Amatucci, and Mr. Cochrane, would amend the insurance laws to include nurses in all health carriers in the state, on a fee-for-service basis. An insurance policy that reimbursed for physicians, psychiatrists, or psychological services would likewise pay for the services of nurses.

Hopefully, such bills will become law in states throughout America.

Existing Third-Party Payment

Sifton explains that Maryland nurse midwives have won direct insurance reimbursement for their nursing care services. These services need not be provided under physician supervision or referral. Maryland's new laws stipulate that all health carriers in the state must offer policyholders the option to use certified nurse midwives. These laws prohibit medical supervision as a requirement for third-party payment. Medicaid payment for nurse midwives was also approved. This law became effective in the summer of 1978.

Strong opposition to direct reimbursement came from Blue Cross and Blue Shield. These organizations see the laws as the beginning of a trend to pay for nonphysician providers and for preventive care.

Washington State requires insurers of state employees to reimburse nurses directly.[12] The State of California has ruled that nurse practitioners and nurse midwives receive the same rate of reimbursement that physicians receive for similar services. The state health plan, Medi-Cal, has adopted this progressive policy. The problem with this plan is that the reimbursement doesn't go directly to the nurses. The payments go to primary care physicians, outpatient clinics, and hospital outpatient departments. Also, physician supervision is required. Apparently, the nurses bill the insurance company, and the physicians, clinics, or hospitals receive the payments. The California Nurses Association feels that reimbursement of this sort is actually useless.[13]

SUMMARY

Professions are a national and public resource. To fulfill their roles, professions must be integrated into the mainstream of national awareness. Inclusion of nurses in fee schedules of health carriers on a fee-for-service basis will raise public consciousness.

Prussin believes that it is safe to assume that a complete National Health Insurance plan will not be enacted prior to the next presidential election. It is also unlikely that any immediate action will be taken on it. Enactment of a mini-National Health Insurance plan to expand Medicare and Medicaid is possible but unlikely before the next presidential election.[14]

There is a definite need for nurses to receive fee-for-service payments, if only to reduce institution overcrowding. When institutions are overcrowded, the staff is in a rush to provide care. The staff often cannot eat meals or take needed breaks, and they must work overtime. This rushing, stress, wear, and tear is unsafe. Accidents occur as a result of it. Overcrowding of institutions, underservice to the public, and underutilization of nurses need to end now.

There is a lot of talk about nurses being quoted for fee-for-service, but as yet, nothing has crystallized from the idea. Nursing needs to adopt an unrelenting approach to changing legislation. As a matter of social policy, programs, benefits, and insurance plans should be geared to clients' needs and not to the needs of insurance companies, bureaucracies, and institutions.

NOTES

1. Earl Ubell, "Unraveling the Mysteries of Health Insurance," *Family Health* 10, no. 10 (October 1978): 22.

2. Elizabeth Wehr, "Carter Lists 'Principles' of National Health Plan," *Congressional Quarterly Weekly Report* 36, no. 31 (August 5, 1978): 2058.

3. Ingeborg G. Mauksch, Ph.D., F.A.A.N., "On National Health Insurance," *American Journal of Nursing* 78, no. 8 (August 1978): 1327.

4. A.J. Vogl, ed., "The Father of Medicare Looks at National Health Insurance," *Medical Economics* (September 5, 1977): 225–6.

5. Elizabeth Wehr, "Senate Defies Carter on Nurse Training Aid," *Congressional Quarterly Weekly Report* 36, no. 24 (June 17, 1978): 1544–5.

6. Martin Donsky, "Nurse Training Aid Veto," *Congressional Quarterly Weekly Report* 36, no. 46 (November 18, 1978): 3323.

7. K. James Skipper, Jr., "Addendum to the Right to Adequate Health Care," *Nursing Digest* 4, no. 1 (January-February 1976): 18.

8. Arnold Birenbaum, "Home Care—An Alternative to the High Cost of Hospitalization," *Intellect* 107 (July 1978): 53.

9. Cathryne A. Welch, "Health Care Distribution and Third-Party Payment for Nurses' Services," *American Journal of Nursing* 75, no. 10 (October 1975): 1844.

10. Raymond J. Donovan, Jr., M.D., "Prescribe Home Care? Now I Can," *Medical Economics* (September 5, 1977): 145, 148, 149, 153.

11. Wolfgang H. Rosenberg, ed., "GAO Reports Home-Health Care Cheaper than Nursing Homes," *Aging* (March-April 1978): 9.

12. David W. Sifton, ed., "Nursing News: Independent Practitioners Win Direct Payment—With No M.D.-Strings Attached," *RN* 41, no. 8 (August 1978): 11.

13. David W. Sifton, ed., "Nursing News: Plan Pays Same Fee for M.D., R.N. Care," *RN* 41, no. 12 (December 1978): 7.

14. Jeffrey A. Prussin, M.A., "National Health Insurance: A Political Issue at the Crossroads," *Nurse Educator* 3, no. 6 (November-December 1978): 27.

Chapter 15

The Challenge

PROFESSIONALISM

Every nurse has potential to be a private nurse practitioner. Nursing has been trying to reach out to the public. The private practice model is one very positive and direct way to achieve greater public accessibility. Nurses should meet this challenge by assuming responsibilities. Private practice can give nursing the added professionalism and professional awareness that it has been seeking. Nurses should band together as a professionally cohesive assemblage to create a united front for the installation of widespread private practice and third-party payment.

New Decisions for Nurses

Effective professionals are people of action; they know how to make decisions and implement them. As more nurses implement private practice and demand third-party payment for their services, a new era in nursing care will come to fruition. This era will produce pride, a major step towards better health care in America. It will be initiated by nurses for the public.

Nursing on a par with primary providers enhances health care. A deeper, more professional nurse-client and nurse-colleague relationship could be realized. These are two major themes in nurses' arguments as they seek greater recognition.

Nursing is an integral part of health care, and advances in nursing must return financial and professional rewards. Nurses know what they need, and they want to perform their roles well. Others should not determine these rewards to nurses solely on the basis of their own awareness of nursing needs and wants. Since nursing is such an integral part of health care, it should take an integral role in third-party reimbursement decision making.

221

Nursing needs to state its roles and functions in health care firmly and clearly. As members of the nursing profession, nurses have an obligation to contribute to the advancement and general welfare of nursing and the public. Independent efforts on the part of some nurses and organized efforts by other nurses will accomplish this goal. The nursing profession must band together to set policy and take stands on issues.

Uustal says the nursing profession is in a state of dynamic redefinition. Nurses are faced with the challenge of redefining their roles and re-examining their values. There is an increased need for nurses to be in touch with clients' needs.[1]

Nurses have been maintaining a dynamic enterprise. The contemporary trend is for nurses to devise their own roles, since no one else knows them better.

The Time is Ripe

Some nurses may feel that the concept of private practice is ahead of its time or that it is grandiose. Neither is true. The time to act is now, while the realization of its need is uppermost in the minds of nurses, colleagues, insurance companies, congresses, and the public. Some nurses have already begun practicing this way; more nurses should begin. Perhaps they are waiting for the go ahead from nursing leaders and authorities. Such leaders and authorities should publicly announce their stand on the issues relating to private nursing practice. Perhaps the American Nurses Association could offer the nurses and public its stand.

Nurses need to make a realistic appraisal of their circumstances. The nursing profession would benefit if nurses were a bit more professionally chauvinistic. If organized nursing were to gain strength like other organizations, it could back a National Health Insurance plan that would enable nurses to enter private practice in more meaningful ways, that would include nurses on a fee-for-service basis and that would cover a vast array of nursing services.

Changes in the public demand nursing care be provided in new ways. The consumer seems to have accepted these changes more readily than nurses themselves. People are becoming more sophisticated, better educated, more inquisitive, more demanding, and more aware of what nurses can do for them. It is time for nursing to enlighten the public as to what approach it will employ to provide added and extended care. Private nursing practice is the most meaningful way to give the public the nursing care it is demanding.

Saba and Skapik point out that a new source of information is available to nurses in the form of a computerized Nursing Information Center (NIC). It operates through the efforts of the Division of Nursing, Bureau of Health Manpower of the Health Resources Administration, U.S. Public Health Service. NIC provides human resource planners with information as a component of the National Health Planning Information Center (NHPIC). One of its many functions is performing computerized searches of information on nursing resources, nurse planning, and resources development practice and methodology.

The NHPIC was established in 1974 under the National Health Planning and Resources Development Act of 1974 (PL 93-641). In this Act, Congress authorized development of a central resource for health planning information. It would have a clearinghouse function to support health planning and resource development.

The NIC is a good place to obtain data related to nursing resources and planning. Its services are available to anyone contacting it.[2] Diligent use of the Nursing Information Center may expedite the widespread use of private nursing practices as health provision centers.

Retired Americans

The American Association of Retired Persons publishes the *AARP News Bulletin.* Articles in this bulletin frequently cite the lack of health care to the elderly. The shortage of health care personnel accessible to the elderly coupled with lack of funding for their health care, are frequent topics. The elderly sorely need the attention that private nurse practitioners can provide, but they are unable to turn to the nurses in their communities because public or private insurance does not cover nurses.

The elderly, a growing and needy community, could benefit if nurses were included in public and private fee schedules on a fee-for-service basis. Nurses could manage around-the-clock health maintenance programs for retirement villages. A nursing practice in a retirement village could provide care to the elderly. Emergency lines to every home or apartment could be provided so the elderly could signal the private nursing practice when an emergency arose, thus ensuring professional aid immediately.

Face Reality

Call it future shock or reality shock, the "future" needs for nursing care are here today. The public puts its hope and faith for the future in today's educational products. Hopefully, nursing graduates and nurses are prepared for today's health care needs. Nurses who are prepared for today's challenges evolve into tomorrow's leaders. Therein lies the future of nursing.

As Blau explains, many people find themselves in emergency departments when they do not have an emergency. True emergencies comprise 20 percent of emergency department visits. The remaining 80 percent are walk-in clients with ordinary medical problems. The emergency department has become the general practitioner, scoring poorly in bedside manner and leaving you waiting for hours. The number of people using emergency departments to replace the waning general practitioner has doubled in the last 15 years. People have nowhere else to turn.[3]

Safron states that a 1971 report prepared by the Department of Health, Education and Welfare said that extending the scope of nursing practice is essential to achieve the goal of equal access to health services for all. The National Joint Practice Commission, an interprofessional organization of the American Medical Association and the American Nurses Association, provided a forum for nurses and physicians to explore ways in which they can work together for the public benefit.[4]

It is time to implement new methods of delivering care. The answer is in small, copious health care centers (private practices) scattered throughout neighborhoods, aided by government incentives, loans, third-party payment, and public recognition.

Spinoffs

Many side effects would occur by large-scale use of private nurse practitioners. Inflation of health care costs, and increased taxes (if nurses were reimbursed by public funds) could be curbed. Disease prevention and treatment would improve, and the public would have an increased availability of health care. Also, problems of transportation to and from health care providers could be reduced if each community had nurse practitioners.

The shortage of physicians would be curtailed if nurses provided primary care. Nurses can teach clients a great deal of health care and visit the homebound. The nursing profession would receive the professional recognition it needs to better provide to the public.

An identity change may occur in the nursing profession also. If nurses provided primary care, children would get an increased exposure and awareness of nursing. They could learn that either sex can enter it and practice truly professional roles, thus adding dignity to the profession. This could increase the numbers of future nurses, as young people make up our future. In effect, the entire public and profession would have an increased identity of what this profession is all about.

As one private nurse practitioner retires, moves out of the area, or expires, another private nurse practitioner could purchase that business or private practice. What he or she would be purchasing is a developed physical location with ready-made clientele.

Check-Off List

Quick reference to what is needed for entry into private practice is included in the following check-off list. Table 15-1 will enable you to quickly review some of the demands of private practice.

Nurses, each and every one who considers entry into private practice, should take stock of their life situation. They should ask what they want to do with their careers, what they want to do for their profession, and what they want their profession to do for them.

Association of Private Nurse Practitioners

An organized alliance of private nurse practitioners could strengthen their ability to fulfill needs and to offer services of the private practitioners and their clients. Readers who wish to become involved in an association for private nurse practitioners should complete the information form in the Appendix and return it to the publisher. You are encouraged to mail additional pertinent data and ask questions. Sending a self-addressed, stamped envelope would prove helpful, since the magnitude of response may be large.

SUMMARY

Nurses need to look to the present, not the future, for reform. What nursing can do now, not what it will do or has done, is the primary way to incorporate private nurse practitioners into present health care systems.

Nurses are clamoring for increased recognition and public service. Entry into private practice and obtaining funds from third parties are the fastest and best ways to achieve this recognition. Fee-for-service quotation is needed for nursing services whether the nurse is employed traditionally or in private practice.

Private practice nursing is primary nursing, since nurses assume responsibility for their clients' care on a continuing basis. Private practice renews the nursing commitment to the client.

Mauksch states that as we look to the year 2000, we need to plan well for health care. This plan needs to be a better one than we have had. There will be about 100 million more people than there are now. In the year 2000 about 80 percent of the population will be urbanized, and 17 percent will be over 65 years of age. If we have not met the health care needs of today, how will we in the year 2000? Careful planning is needed now.[5]

Jennings points out that there is agreement that present health care leaves a lot to be desired. Accessibility of services is a top priority and a sensitive issue

Table 15-1 Private Practice Check-Off List

1. Personal preparation
   a. Self-evaluation, self-awareness, self-discipline, and self-confidence
   b. Self-study
   c. Continuing education
   d. Competence in nursing
   e. Counteracting false assumptions for reality of private practice
   f. Ethical considerations
   g. Finances
   h. Managerial and administrative skills
   i. Traditional employment
   j. Willingness to accept the responsibility
2. Legal considerations
   a. Local ordinances
   b. State laws
   c. Legal counsel of attorney
   d. Counsel of accountant
   e. Malpractice insurance
3. Community needs
   a. Physicians' questionnaire
   b. Hours
   c. Consultations
   d. Community assessment
4. Private practice
   a. Location
   b. Type of services
   c. Group or single practice
   d. Employees
   e. Organizational chart
   f. Layout
   g. Equipment
   h. Fee schedules
5. Professional relations
   a. Letters of introduction
   b. Telephone book advertisement
   c. Consultations
6. Safety mechanisms
   a. Nurses' records
   b. Physicians' orders
   c. Assistance as needed
   d. Collaboration

e. Awareness of limitations
f. The nursing process

---

for consumers. People want quick, close, complete health care. The lack of easily accessible health care is a sore spot in the present health care system. Third-party payment could enable nurses to demand adequate nurse-client ratios for the safe delivery of quality care.[6]

Schorr says that forecasts for 1982 show that more nurses will be needed, particularly nurses prepared at the bachelor's, master's, and doctoral levels, for work in hospitals, schools, and nursing homes. This forecast is a result of the study by Western Interstate Commission for Higher Education. More nurses are needed for all areas; the community was a special area cited.[7]

Nursing needs to increase the care offered to the public. This care should be provided in a way acceptable and desirable to the public and manageable to nursing. Private practice nursing is one answer.

The fact that many nurses have taken the initiative to enter private practice is consensual validation for any nurse considering private nursing practice. Private nurse practitioners with the courage of their convictions have paved the way for other nurses to follow. The fact that they have published articles, met clients' needs, and practiced ethically demonstrates to their peers the value of practicing nursing privately.

Legislative attempts to include nurses in health carriers' fee schedules for fee-for-service reimbursement constitutes political proof of the public need and the credibility of nurses through the legislative eye. The reason the bills have not become law are not lack of credibility but lack of nursing's clout to support the proposed bills through the procedure of lawmaking.

Thus, nurses are faced with the challenge of a new, innovative health care mechanism as we enter the 1980's. Nurses can unite to provide services to alleviate the crowded, uncomfortable, and sometimes uncompassionate care that many people currently receive. We *can* provide quality, professional, and realistic health care through private nursing practices.

NOTES

1. Diane B. Uustal, R.N., M.S., "Values Clarification in Nursing: Application to Practice," *American Journal of Nursing* 78, no. 12 (December 1978): 2058.

2. Virginia K. Saba, M.A., M.S., and Kathleen A. Skapik, M.A., "Nursing Information Center," *American Journal of Nursing* 79, no. 1 (January 1979): 86-7.

3. Melinda Blau, "Emergency!" *New York* 11, no. 8 (February 20, 1978): 39–40.

4. Claire Safron, "Their Patients Call them Super-Nurses," *Today's Health* (July-August 1975): 21.

5. Ingeborg G. Mauksch, R.N., "Paradox of Risk Takers," *AORN Journal* 25, no. 7 (June 1977): 1289, 1292.

6. Carole P. Jennings, R.N., M.A., "Nursing's Case for Third-Party Reimbursement," *American Journal of Nursing* 79, no. 1 (January 1979): 111.

7. Thelma M. Schorr, ed., "News: WICHE Predicts Increased Nurse Needs in Hospitals, Schools, Nursing Homes," *American Journal of Nursing* 78, no. 8 (August 1978): 1286.

State-by-State Summary of Nurse Practice Acts*

*Adopted from Virginia C. Hall, "Summary of Statutory Provisions Governing Legal Scope of Nursing Practice in the Various States," in *The New Health Professionals,* A. Bliss and E. Cohen, eds. (Germantown, Md.: Aspen Systems Corporation, 1977). Reprinted with permission. ©1977 Aspen Systems Corporation.

If Additional Acts Amendment, Criteria and Conditions Stated

State	Type of Definition	Definition Includes Prohibition Against Acts of Diagnosis and Prescription	Rules and Regulations	Professional Opinion	Education and Training	If New Definition, Incorporated some or all of New York's	Prohibitions of Practice of Medicine in Nurse Practice Act	Exception for Nursing in Medical Practice Act	Physician Supervision of Nurse Practitioners	Degree of Supervision
Alabama	New & Additional Acts Amendment	No	Yes	—	—	Yes	No	No	Required for Nurse Anesthetist	Direct for 30 days, then protocol for midwife
Alaska	Traditional & Additional Acts Amendment	Yes (Applies to "medical" acts only and additional acts not subject to prohibition.)	Yes*	—	—	—	No	No	Collaborative relationship for Nurse-Midwife	
Arizona	Traditional & Additional Acts Amendment†	No	Yes*	Yes*	Yes	—	No	Yes (Under physician supervision)	Under direction of and in collaboration with	Presence required for Nurse Anesthetist
Arkansas	Traditional	Yes (Applies to "medical" acts only)	—	—	—	—	No	Yes (Also separate exemption for nurse acting under physician supervision)	Required for Nurse Anesthetist	Presence required
California	New	No	—	—	—	No	No	Yes (For persons lawfully practicing another profession)		As defined by policies and protocols developed for specific setting
Colorado	New & Additional Acts Amendment	No	Yes**	No	Yes	Yes	No	Yes (Also separate exemption for persons acting under physician supervision)	Required	Defined in protocols

State	Definition								
Connecticut	New	No	—	—	—	Yes	Yes	Yes (Under physician supervision)	Not stated
Delaware	Traditional	Yes	—	—	—	—	No	No	Not stated
District of Columbia	No Definition	—	—	—	—	—	No	Yes	Not stated
Florida	Traditional & Additional Acts Amendment	No	Yes	—	—	—	Yes	Yes (Under physician supervision)	Not stated
Georgia	Traditional	No	—	—	—	—	No	Yes (Also separate exemption for persons acting under physician supervision)	Nurse Anesthetists function under direction of physician
Hawaii	Traditional	Yes (Applies to "medical" acts only)	—	—	—	—	No	No (?)[2]	No specific legislation
Idaho	Traditional & Additional Acts Amendment	Yes	Yes (Applies to "medical" acts only and additional acts not subject to prohibition)	No	No	—	No	No	None referred to but "practice policies" for individuals may so indicate
Illinois	Traditional	Yes (Applies to "medical" acts only)	—	—	—	—	No	Yes (For persons lawfully practicing another profession)	No specific legislation
Indiana	New & Additional Acts Amendment	No	Yes***	No	No	Yes	No	Yes	Required for Nurse Anesthetist
Iowa	New & Additional Acts Amendment	No	—	—	—	Yes	Yes	Yes	No specific regulations
Kansas	Traditional	Yes	—	—	—	—	No	Yes (Also separate exemption for persons acting under physician supervision)	No legislation
Kentucky	Traditional	Yes (Applies to "medical" acts only)	—	—	—	—	No	Yes	No legislation
Louisiana	New & Additional Amendment Act	Yes	Yes	—	—	Yes	No	Yes	Required

If Additional Acts Amendment, Criteria and Conditions Stated

State	Type of Definition	Definition Includes Prohibition Against Acts of Diagnosis and Prescription	Rules and Regulations	Professional Opinion	Education and Training	If New Definition, Incorporated some or all of New York's	Prohibitions of Practice of Medicine in Nurse Practice Act	Exception for Nursing in Medical Practice Act	Physician Supervision of Nurse Practitioners	Degree of Supervision
Maine	Traditional & Additional Acts Amendment	No	No	No	Yes	–	No	No	Physician can delegate certain services	
Maryland	New & Additional Acts Amendment	No	Yes**	Yes*	Yes	Yes	No	Yes (For persons lawfully practicing another profession)	Not stated	
Massachusetts	Traditional & Additional Acts Amendment	No	Yes*	Yes**	Yes	Yes	No	Yes (Applies only to nurses performing "Additional acts")	No regulations	
Michigan	Traditional	Yes (Applies to "medical" acts only)	–	–	–	–	No	Yes (For persons lawfully practicing another profession and separate exemption for persons acting under physician supervision)	No specific legislation	
Minnesota	New	No	–	–	–	Yes	No	Yes (For persons lawfully practicing another profession)	No specific legislation	
Mississippi	Traditional & Additional Acts Amendent	Yes (Applies to "medical" acts only and additional acts not subjected to prohibition)	Yes*	No	No	–	No	No	Not stated	

State										
Missouri	New	No	—	—	—	Yes	No	Yes	No specific legislation	
Montana	Traditional	Yes	—	—	—	—	No	Yes	No specific legislation	
Nebraska	New & Additional Amendment Act	Yes, Medicine	Yes	—	—	Yes	No	Yes (For persons lawfully practicing another profession—not applicable to prescription or administration of drugs)	Required	Specific to each approved expanded role
Nevada	Traditional & Additional Acts Amendment	Yes (Applies to "medical" acts only and additional acts not subject to prohibition)	Yes**	Yes*	Yes	—	No	Yes	Collaboration	As agreed in writing
New Hampshire	New & Additional Acts Amendment	Yes (Additional acts not subject to prohibition)	Yes*	Yes**	Yes	Yes	No	Yes	Collaboration	Nurse anesthetists function within physical presence of physician
New Jersey	New	No	—	—	—	Yes	No	Yes (Under physician supervision)	No specific legislation	
New Mexico	Traditional	Yes (Applies to "medical" acts only)	—	—	—	—	No	Yes (Plus separate exemption for nurse practitioners in certain settings)	Required	
New York	New	No	—	—	—	Yes	Yes	Yes (For persons lawfully practicing another profession)	No regulations	
North Carolina	Traditional & Additional Acts Amendment	Yes (Applies to "medical" acts only and excepts acts under supervision of physician)	Yes*	No	—	—	No	Yes (For nursing and those acts "otherwise constituting medical practice" which are permitted by regulations of medical and nursing boards)	Required	Telecommunications, predetermined plan, for emergencies, review of practice
North Dakota	Traditional	No	—	—	—	—	No	No	No regulations	

If Additional Acts Amendment, Criteria and Conditions Stated

State	Type of Definition	Definition Includes Prohibition Against Acts of Diagnosis and Prescription	Rules and Regulations	Professional Opinion	Education and Training	If New Definition, Incorporated some or all of New York's Prohibitions of Practice of Medicine in Nurse Practice Act	Exception for Nursing in Medical Practice Act	Physician Supervision of Nurse Practitioners	Degree of Supervision
Ohio	Traditional	Yes (Applies to "medical" acts only)	—	—	—	—	Yes	Yes (For nurse anesthetists only, under physician supervision)	Required for nurse-midwife and nurse anesthetist	Nurse anesthetist must work in presence of physician
Oklahoma	Traditional	Yes	—	—	—	—	No	Yes (Under physician supervision)	No regulations	
Oregon	New & Additional Acts Amendment	No	Yes**	Yes*	Yes	Yes	No	Yes	Collaboration	
Pennsylvania	New & Additional Acts Amendment	Yes (Applies to "medical" acts only and additional acts not subject to prohibition)	Yes*	No	No	Yes	Yes	No	Required	Telecommunications, predetermined plan for emergency
Rhode Island	Traditional	No	—	—	—	—	No	No	No specific legislation	
South Carolina	Traditional	Yes (Applies to "medical" acts only)	Yes	—	—	—	No	Yes	Required	Near proximity, available for consultation

South Dakota	New & Additional Acts Amendment	No	Yes	No	Yes	Yes	Yes	Yes	Not stated
Tennessee	Traditional	Yes (Applies to "medical" acts only)	—	—	—	—	No	Yes (Plus separate exemption for nurses under physician supervision)	Required	As indicated in written protocols for specific situations
Texas	Traditional	Yes (Applies to "medical" acts only)	Yes	—	—	—	Yes	Yes	Required (for medical treatment)
Utah	New & Additional Acts Amendment	No	—	—	—	Yes	No	Yes	Required
Vermont	New & Additional Acts Amendment	Yes	No	Yes	Yes	Yes	Yes	Yes (Under physician supervision)	No regulations
Virginia	Traditional (Additional Amendments to Medical Practice Act)	No	Yes	—	—	—	No	Yes (Includes specific reference to certain procedures, which must be performed under orders of physician, plus separate exemption for nurses acting under physician supervision pursuant to rules and regulations of Boards of Nursing and Medicine)	Must be available for consultation
Washington	New & Additional Acts Amendment	No	Yes**	Yes*	Yes	Yes	No	No	Uses "scope of practice" as in statements by national associations

If Additional Acts Amendment, Criteria and Conditions Stated

State	Type of Definition	Definition Includes Prohibition Against Acts of Diagnosis and Prescription	Rules and Regulations	Professional Opinion	Education and Training	If New Definition, Incorporated some or all of New York's	Prohibitions of Practice of Medicine in Nurse Practice Act	Exception for Nursing in Medical Practice Act	Physician Supervision of Nurse Practitioners	Degree of Supervision
West Virginia	Traditional	No	—	—	—	—	No	Yes	Required	Nurse anesthetists in presence of physician, nurse-midwives according to ACNM standards
Wisconsin	Traditional	No	—	—	—	—	No	Yes (Under physician supervision)[4]	No specific legislation	
Wyoming	New	No	—	—	—	—	No	Yes (Under physician supervision)	Required	Telecommunications, referral and consultation, regular chart review, predetermined plan for emergencies, protocols for medication

[1] Arizona's additional acts amendment, unlike any other, describes substantively one such act: the dispensing of prepackaged, labelled drugs under certain limited, specific circumstances.

[2] Hawaii has a delegation provision which applies to "any physician-support personnel" and which could be construed as including nurses.

[3] Although Maryland's additional acts amendment does not mention physician supervision, the amendment could be interpreted as subordinate to the definition's general description of nursing as consisting of "independent" nursing functions and "delegated" medical functions, in which case any medical acts within the additional acts amendment would have to be delegated acts.

[4] North Carolina's additional acts amendment does not mention physician supervision, but it appears in a separate section from the definition and would appear to be subordinate to that provision of the definition which prohibits acts of medical diagnosis and prescription except under physician supervision.

[5] Oregon alone among the states with additional acts amendments which refer to professional opinion speaks only of nursing opinion, as opposed to medical and nursing opinion.

[6] Wisconsin's law in this regard is somewhat oblique, but it would appear that not only nurses but any persons are authorized to "assist" physicians.

*By Boards of Nursing and Medicine.

**By Board of Nursing.

***By Board of Nursing or "in collaboration with" Board of Medicine.

*Cumulative with rules and regulations.

**Independent of rules and regulations.

Selected Bibliography

Abdellah, Faye G., Ph.D. "Nurse Practitioners and Nursing Practice." *American Journal of Public Health* 66:245–6.

Aday, Liv Ann, Ph.D.; Andersen, Ronald, Ph.D.; and Anderson, Odin W., Ph.D. "Social Surveys and Health Policy—Implications for National Health Insurance." *Public Health Reports* 92: 508-17.

Aeschliman, Dorothy D., R.N., M.S. "A Strategy for Change." *Nurse Practitioner* 1: 121–124.

Agree, Betty C. "Beginning an Independent Nursing Practice." *American Journal of Nursing* 74: 636–642.

Alexander, Edythe. *Nursing Administration in the Hospital Health Care System.* Saint Louis: The C. V. Mosby Company, 1972.

Alexander, Linda, Ph.D. "The Nurse Practitioner and Professional Growth." *Nurse Practitioner* 1: 32–33.

Alford, Dolores Marsh, R.N., M.S.N. and Jensen, Janet Moll, R.N., B.S.N. "Reflections on Private Practice." *American Journal of Nursing* 76: 1966–1968.

Allen, Louis L. *Starting and Succeeding in Your Own Small Business.* New York: Grosset and Dunlap, 1968.

American Board of Medical Specialties. *Directory of Medical Specialists,* 18th ed. Chicago, Illinois: Marquis Who's Who, Inc., 1977.

Arndt, Clara, R.N., M.S. and Huckabay, Loucine Daderian M., R.N., B.S., M.S., Ph.D. *Nursing Administration.* Saint Louis: The C. V. Mosby Company, 1975.

Atkinson, William. "You Can Be an Effective Supervisor." *Nursing Care* 10: 22–24, 31.

Bakdash, Diane P., R.N., M.N. "Become an Assertive Nurse." *American Journal of Nursing* 78: 1710–12.

Battersby, Mark E. "Year-End Tax Savings for Nurses." *Nursing Care* 9: 19–20.

Beason, Cathy, ed. "Nurse Practitioners: The Flak from Doctors is Getting Heavier." *RN* 41: 27–37.

Belote, Martha. "Four Nurses Hang Out a Shingle." *American Journal of Nursing* 72: 1782.

Bennett, Addison C. "Education and Training Need to be Brought Up-To-Date." *Hospitals JAHA* 52: 75–6, 84.

Benson, Evelyn Rose, R.N., M.P.H. and McDevitt, Joan Quinn, R.N., M.S.N. *Community Health and Nursing Practice.* Englewood Cliffs, New Jersey: Prentice-Hall, Inc., 1976.

Berg, Donald L., ed. "Cartercare: What You Can Expect and When." *RN* 41: 72–74, 78, 80, 82, 87–8.

Birenbaum, Arnold. "Home Care—An Alternative to the High Cost of Hospitalization." *Intellect* 107: 52–54.

Blau, Melinda. "Emergency." *New York* 11: 39–40.

Bowman, Rosemary A. and Culpepper, Rebecca C. "National Health Insurance: Some of the Issues." *American Journal of Nursing* 75: 2017–2021.

Boyd, Nora. "New Help for PCs: Physicians' Spouses." *Physicians Management* 17: 31–32.

Branson, Helen Kitchen, R.N., M.A. "A New Nurse for the New Health Care." *Nursing Care* 10: 28–29.

Brickner, Philip W.; Bolger, Anne G.; Boyle, Sister Mary T.; Duque, Sister Teresita; Holland, Patricia; Janeski, James F.; Kaufman, Arthur; Madden, Patricia M. "Outreach to Welfare Hotels, the Homebound, the Frail." *American Journal of Nursing* 76: 762–764.

Britton, Ann H. "Rights to Privacy in Medical Records." *The Journal of Legal Medicine* 3: 24–31.

Brock, Leah. "Salaries in Community Health Agencies—1978." *Nursing Outlook* 26: 772–776.

Brown, Esther Lucile, Ph.D. *Nursing Reconsidered: A Study of Change.* Philadelphia: J. B. Lippincott Company, 1971.

Bullough, Bonnie. "Influences on Role Expansion." *American Journal of Nursing* 76: 1476–1481.

Burke, Ronald J., Ph.D. and Goodale, James G., Ph.D. "New Way to Rate Nurse Performance." *Hospitals JAHA* 47: 62, 64–65, 68.

Burke, William J. and Zaloon, Basil J. *Blueprint for Professional Service Corporations.* New York: Thomas T. Crowell Company, 1970.

Cazalas, Mary W., R.N., J.D. *Nursing and the Law,* 3rd ed. Germantown, Maryland: Aspen Systems Corporation, 1978.

Choniski, Carol, R.N.; Hamer, Carol, R.N.; Hamm, Sally, R.N.; McDonald, Mabel, R.N.; and Nelson, Patricia, R.N. "Playing With the Entry Requirement: A Game We Can't Afford." *RN* 41: 27–8, 30, 32.

Christman, Luther. "Accountability and Autonomy are More Than Rhetoric." *Nurse Educator* 3: 3–6.

Churchill, Larry. "Ethical Issues of a Profession in Transition." *American Journal of Nursing* 77: 873–875.

Close, Henry T. "On Saying NO to People: A Pastoral Letter." *Journal of Nursing Digest* 3: 49–52.

Collins, Verla. "1977—The Year of the Nurse." *Vital Speeches of the Day* 43: 590–3.

Cook, Harvey R. *Selecting Advertising Media: A Guide for Small Business.* Washington, D.C.: Small Business Administration, 1969.

Cooper, James K., M.D. "No-Fault Malpractice Insurance: Swedish Plan Shows Us the Way." *Hospitals JAHA* 52:115–6, 118, 120.

Cummings, Dana, R.N., B.S. "What a Rural FNP Needs to Know." *American Journal of Nursing* 78: 1332–1333.

Cunningham, Robert M., Jr. "NHI: A Matter of Degree." *Hospitals JAHA* 52: 64–7.

Curran, Connie L. "What Kind of Continuing Education?" *Supervisor Nurse* 8: 72–75.

Cutler, M. J. "Nursing Leadership and Management: An Historical Perspective." *Nursing Administrative Quarterly* 1:7–19.

Daubert, Elizabeth A., R.N., M.P.H. "A System to Evaluate Home Health Care Services." *Nursing Outlook* 25: 168–171.

Donnelly, Gloria Ferraro, R.N., M.S.N. "How to Soothe a Savage Surgeon." *RN* 41: 45–47.

Donovan, Hedley, ed. "Private-Practice Nurses." *Time,* March 12, 1973, p. 70.

Donovan, Helen M., R.N., M.A. *Nursing Service Administration Managing the Enterprise.* Saint Louis: The C. V. Mosby Company, 1975.

Donovan, Raymond J., Jr., M.D. "Prescribe Home Care? Now I Can." *Medical Economics,* September 5, 1977, pp. 145–153.

Donsky, Martin. "Nurse Training Aid Veto." *Congressional Quarterly Weekly Report* 36: 3323.

Douglass, Mae Laura, R.N., B.A., M.S. and Beirs, Olivia Em, R.N., B.S., M.A. *Nursing Leadership in Action.* St. Louis: The C. V. Mosby Company, 1974.

Duffy, Kay M., R.N. "Changing Behavior: A Fun Approach That Works." *RN* 41: 103–104.

Ellis, Barbara. "Nursing Profession Undergoes Intensive Scrutiny and Adjustment." *Hospitals JAHA* 51: 139–144.

Emkey, Kenneth, M.D. "Tempering the Turmoil of an Office Emergency." *Nursing 77* 7: 16–20.

Epstein, Rhoda B. "Focus on Nursing Education." *Proceedings—Open Curriculum Conference IV.* New York: National League for Nursing, September 22–23, 1975.

Fair, Thelma. "Self-Education: Don't Let It Stop." *Nursing Care* 9: 15.

Faris, June B., ed. "Survey Shows Medicaid Money is Misspent." *Aging,* August, 1977, p. 32.

Flanagan, Patrick, ed. "Are Physicians More or Less Respected Today?" *Physician's Management* 17: 59–63.

Flanagan, Patrick, ed. "Office Collection Procedures." *Physician's Management* 17: 15–16.

Fromm, Linda. "The Problem in Nursing: Nurses!" *Supervisor Nurse* 8: 15–16.

Ganong, Joan M., R.N., M.S. and Ganong, Warren L., C.M.C. *Nursing Management.* Germantown, Maryland: Aspen Systems Corporation, 1976.

Gavin, Marshall. "Consumer Services: Inhospital Reachout." *Hospitals JAHA* 49: 65–67.

Geyman, John P., M.D.; Brown, Thomas C., Ph.D.; and Rivers, Kevin, A.B. "Referrals in Family Practice: A Comparative Study by Geographic Region and Practice Setting." *The Journal of Family Practice* 3: 163–167.

Gill, Sandra L. "Leadership Guidelines for Decision Making." *Imprint* 25: 48–49, 69, 70, 72.

Gillette, Paul J., Ph.D. " 'The Screwing of the Average Man.' " *Modern Medicine* 43: 23–27.

Goodspeed, Harriett E. "The Independent Practitioner—Can It Survive?" *Journal of Psychiatric Nursing and Mental Health Services* 14: 33–34.

Greighton, Helen, R.N., B.S.N., A.B., A.M., M.S.N., J.D. *Law Every Nurse Should Know,* 3rd ed. Philadelphia: W. B. Saunders Company, 1975.

Grissum, Marlene, R.N., M.S. "How You Can Become a Risk-Taker and a Role-Breaker." *Nursing 76* 6: 89–98.

Haase, Patricia T. "Pathways to Practice—Part I." *American Journal of Nursing* 76: 806–809.

Hankin, Robert A. "Why America Must Have National Health Insurance." *Intellect* 105: 340.

"Health Plan Order." *Congressional Quarterly Weekly Report* 36: 2059.

"Health Policy: Congress Overrides Health Services Veto." *Congressional Quarterly Almanac,* 1975, pp. 591–599.

"Health Policy: Medicare Hearings." *Congressional Quarterly Almanac,* 1975, pp. 615–620.

Hedrich, Vivian, M.A., "A National Survey: Educating for the Expanded Role." *Nurse Practitioner* 3: 13–16.

Hein, Eleanor, R.N., M.S. and Leavitt, Maribelle, R.N., M.S. "Providing Emotional Support to Patients." *Nursing 77* 7: 39–41.

Henderson, Betty, R.N., M.N. "Nursing Diagnosis: Theory and Practice." *Advances in Nursing Science* 1: 75–83.

Hershey, Nathan. "Physician Reaction to Quality of Care Assessment by Nurses." *The Hospital Medical Staff* 5: 9–12.

Hollowell, Edward E. "What Every Nurse Should Know About Tort Liability." *Hospitals JAHA* 51: 97–8, 100.

Hopper, Susan. "Becoming an Administrator Overnight!" *Nursing Outlook* 23: 752–754.

Horsley, Jack E., J.D. "When to 'Tattle' on Physician Misconduct," *RN* 41: 17, 22, 24.

"House Committee Scraps President's Hospital Cost Control Proposal." *Congressional Quarterly Weekly Report* 36: 1885–7.

Howard, Ernest B., M.D. *American Medical Directory, Geographical Register of Physicians,* 26th ed. Chicago, Illinois: American Medical Association, 1974.

Jennings, Carole P., R.N., M.A. "Nursing's Case for Third-Party Reimbursement." *American Journal of Nursing* 79: 111–114.

Jones, Susan L., R.N., Ph.D. and Jones, Paul K., Ph.D. "Nursing Student Definitions of the 'Real' Nurse." *Journal of Nursing Education* 16: 15–21.

Jordan, Clifford A., R.N., Ed.D. "Accountability for Nursing Practice," *AORN Journal* 27: 1076–1080.

Kaplan, Sanford A., M.D. "How to Disentangle Yourself from the Sticky Web of Bureaucracy." *Modern Medicine* 43: 79, 81–2, 84.

Keeling, Arlene W. and Noriega, Lawrence. "Continuing Education—Independently!" *Supervisor Nurse* 9: 45–51.

Kelly, Nancy Perpall, R.N., B.S. "Taking the Errors Out of Phone Orders." *Nursing 78* 8: 19–20.

Kinlein, Lucille M. "Independent Nurse Practitioner." *Nursing Outlook* 20: 22–24.

Knafl, Kathleen Astin. "How Nurse Practitioner Students Confuse Their 'Role.'" *Nursing Outlook* 26: 650–653.

Koltz, Charles J., Jr., R.N., B.S.N., "Private Practice: A Nurse's Challenge." *Point of View* 13: 17–19.

Kramer, Marlene. *Reality Shock: Why Nurses Leave Nursing.* Saint Louis: The C. V. Mosby Company, 1974.

Kron, Thora, R.N., B.S. "How to Become a Better Leader." *Nursing 76* 6: 67–83.

Kruzas, Anthony T. *Medical and Health Information Directory.* Detroit, Michigan: Gale Research Co., 1977.

Kuba, Anna, R.N. "National Trends in Licensing Laws." *Texas Nursing,* June 1976, pp. 7–8, 10.

Laukhuf, Jean Kast, R.N. "How a 21-Year-Old Director of Nursing Almost Blew It." *RN* 41: 99–101.

Lenburg, C. B. "Bicentennial Forecast: Nursing Education." *RN* 39: 21–2, 28, 30.

Lesly, Philip. *Public Relations Handbook,* 3rd ed. Englewood Cliffs, N.J.: Prentice-Hall, Inc., 1967.

Lesly, Philip. *Lesly's Public Relations Handbook.* Englewood Cliffs, N.J.: Prentice-Hall, Inc., 1971.

Levine, E. Myra. "Nursing Ethics and the Ethical Nurse." *American Journal of Nursing* 77: 845–849.

Lewis, Charles E., M.D., Sc.D. and Cheyovich, Therese K., R.N., M.S. "Who is a Nurse Practitioner? Processes of Care and Patients' and Physicians' Perceptions." *Medical Care* 14: 365–371.

Linn, Lawrence S., Ph.D. "Patient Acceptance of the Family Nurse Practitioner." *Medical Care* 14: 357–364.

Linn, Lawrence S., Ph.D. "Type of Nursing Education and the Nurse Practitioner Experience." *Nurse Practitioner* 1: 28–33.

Little, Marilyn, B.S., M.A. "Physicians' Attitudes Toward Employment of Nurse Practitioners." *Nurse Practitioner* 3: 26, 28–9.

Lively, Carol A. "P.L. 93–641: A Recipe for Action." *Hospitals JAHA* 52: 65–68, 124.

Lynaugh, E. Joan and Bates, Barbara. "The Two Languages of Nursing and Medicine." *American Journal of Nursing* 73: 66–69.

Lyons, Thomas. "Role Clarity, Need for Clarity, Satisfaction, Tension, and Withdrawal." *Organizational Behavior and Human Performance* 6: 99–110.

Maas, M.; Specht, J.; and Jacox, A. "Nurse Autonomy, Reality Not Rhetoric." *American Journal of Nursing* 75: 2201–2208.

McAtee, Patricia Rooney, R.N. and Silver, Henry K., M.D. "What About a National Nurse-Practitioner Program?" *RN* 38: 22–27.

McClure, Margaret L., R.N., Ed.D. "The Long Road to Accountability." *Nursing Outlook* 26: 47–50.

McShane, Nancy Gerberding, R.N., M.S.N. and Smith, Elizabeth McDowell, R.N., M.A. "Starting a Private Practice in Mental Health Nursing." *American Journal of Nursing* 78: 2050–2070.

Marshall, Eliot. "On the Hill: Healthy Skepticism." *The New Republic,* April 29, 1978, pp. 10–12.

Mauksch, Ingeborg G. "Nursing is Coming of Age Through the Practitioner Movement." *American Journal of Nursing* 75: 1834–1843.

Mauksch, Ingeborg G., Ph.D., F.A.A.N. "On National Health Insurance." *American Journal of Nursing* 78: 1322–7.

Mauksch, Ingeborg G. "Paradox of Risk Takers." *AORN Journal* 25: 1289–1312.

Mauldin, Brenda C., R.N. "Professional Work Rates Professional Pay." *RN* 41: 43.

Marriner, Ann, R.N., Ph.D. *The Nursing Process.* Saint Louis: The C. V. Mosby Company, 1975.

Martin, Morgan, M.D. "The Bureaucrat—The Taming of the DHEW." *JAMA* 223: 976–8.

"Medical Peer Review." *Congressional Quarterly Almanac,* 1974, p. 376.

Meyer, Linn. "Educational Requirements Raise Controversy for Health Personnel." *Hospitals JAHA* 51: 119–125.

Miller, Harriet. "Rural Elderly Face Shortage of Doctors; Medicare Aid Needed." *AARP News Bulletin* 18:6.

Moniz, Donna, R.N., M.N. "Putting Assertiveness Techniques into Practice." *American Journal of Nursing* 78: 1713.

Montange, Charles H., J.D. "Consumer Protection and Professional Services." *The Journal of Legal Medicine* 4: 23–27.

"More Home Health Care for Aged Patients Voted." *Congressional Quarterly Weekly Report* 34: 2544–5.

Murchison, Irene, R.N., B.S., M.A.; Nicholas, Thomas S., A.B., M.S., LL.B.; and Hanson, Rachel, R.N., B.S., M.S. *Legal Accountability in the Nursing Process.* Saint Louis: The C. V. Mosby Company, 1978.

Murray, Ruth, R.N., M.S.N. and Zentner, Judith, R.N., M.A. *Nursing Concepts for Health Promotion.* Englewood Cliffs, N.J.: Prentice-Hall, Inc., 1975.

Nassau-Suffolk Health Systems Agency, Inc. *Annual Implementation Plan for Nassau-Suffolk.* Melville, New York: 1978.

Nassau-Suffolk Health Systems Agency, Inc. *Health Systems Plan 1978 Summary.* Melville, New York: 1978.

Nordberg, Beatrice and King, Lynelle. "Third-Party Payment for Patient Education." *American Journal of Nursing* 76: 1269–1271.

Pattison, E. M. "Residency Training in Community Psychiatry." *American Journal of Psychiatry* 128: 1097–1102.

"Peer Review." *Congressional Quarterly Almanac,* 1974, pp. 431–2.

Pesznecker, Betty, R.N., M.S. "Life Change: A Challenge for Nurse Practitioners." *Nurse Practitioner* 1: 21–25.

Petrof, John V.; Carusone, Peter S.; and McDavid, John E. *Small Business Management: Concepts and Techniques for Improving Decisions.* New York, N.Y.: McGraw-Hill Book Company, 1972.

Presser, Carole S. "Factors Affecting the Geographic Distribution of Physicians." *The Journal of Legal Medicine* 3: 12–18.

Prussin, Jeffrey A., M.A. "National Health Insurance: A Political Issue at the Crossroads." *Nurse Educator* 3: 23–7.

"Public Laws." *Congressional Quarterly Almanac,* 1972, p. 1145.

Ramphal, Marjorie. "Peer Review." *American Journal of Nursing* 74: 63–87.

Randolph, Gretchen T. "Experiences in Private Practice." *Journal of Psychiatric Nursing and Mental Health Services* 13: 16–19.

Regan, William Andrew, J.D. "How Do You Expose an Errant M.D.?—Very, Very Carefully!" *RN* 41: 39–40.

Reinhardt, Adina M. and Quinn, Mildred D. *Family-Centered Community Nursing.* Saint Louis: The C. V. Mosby Company, 1973.

Reschke, Elaine M., R.N. "It's Easy to Collect Fees at Time of Treatment." *Physician's Management* 17: 9–11, 13–14.

Rodin, Rita. "Today's Florence Nightingales Everything's Changed but the Idealism." *Working Woman* 3: 31–35.

Roovers, G. T. "Pluses and Minuses Computerized Billing in Private Practice." *Physician's Management* 17: 17–21.

Rosasco, Louise C., R.N. "Of Nursing Practice and Nurse Practitioners." *Nursing Digest,* May-June, 1975, pp. 36–37.

Rosenberg, Wolfgang H., ed. "GAO Reports Home-Health Care Cheaper than Nursing Homes." *Aging,* March-April 1978, p. 9.

Rothman, Daniel A., J.D. and Rothman, Lloyd Nancy, R.N., B.S.N., M.Ed. *The Professional Nurse and the Law.* Boston: Little, Brown and Company, 1977.

Roy, Sister Callista and Obloy, Sister Marcia. "The Practitioner Movement— Toward a Science of Nursing." *American Journal of Nursing* 78: 1698–1702.

"Rural Health Clinics." *Congressional Quarterly Almanac,* 1977, pp. 515–7.

Saba, Virginia K., M.A., M.S. and Skapik, Kathleen A., M.A. "Nursing Information Center." *American Journal of Nursing* 79: 86–7.

Sadler, Alfred M., Jr., M.D. "New Health Practitioner Education: Problems and Issues." *Journal of Medical Education.* 50: 67–73.

Safron, Claire. "Their Patients Call Them Supernurses." *Today's Health,* July-August 1975, pp. 20–51.

Sargis, Nancy M., R.N., Ed.D. "Will Nursing Directors' Attitudes Affect Future Collective Bargaining?" *Journal of Nursing Administration* 8: 21–6.

Sateren, Judith L. and Westover, Devra E. "Baccalaureate Preparation for Action-Practice Nursing." *Nurse Educator* 3: 12–14.

Schlotfeldt, Rozella, R.N., Ph.D., F.A.A.N. "Rozella Schlotfeldt Says." *American Journal of Nursing* 76, no. 1: 105–107.

Schorr, Thelma M., R.N. "ANA Convention '76." *American Journal of Nursing* 76: 1123–1138.

Schorr, Thelma M., R.N. "Meeting in Minneapolis." *American Journal of Nursing* 73: 1198–1206.

Schorr, Thelma M., R.N., ed. "News: WICHE Predicts Increased Nurse Needs in Hospitals, Schools, Nursing Homes." *American Journal of Nursing* 78: 1286.

Schrader, Elinor S., ed. "Can Nurses Communicate Directly with Physicians?" *AORN Journal* 28: 193–194.

Schrader, Elinor S., ed. "Direct Reimbursement for Nursing Involves Roles, Certification!" *AORN Journal* 25: 843–4, 846.

Schrader, Elinor S., ed. "Reimbursement for Nursing Services in Rural Clinics." *AORN Journal* 25: 846.

Schweitzer, Stuart O., Ph.D. and Record, Cassela Jane, Ph.D. "Third-Party Payments for New Health Professionals: An Alternative to Fractional Reimbursement in Outpatient Care." *Public Health Reports* 92: 518–526.

"Senate Passes Measure Consolidating and Extending Programs for Elderly." *Congressional Quarterly Weekly Report* 36: 2211–13.

Sifton, David W., ed. "Nursing News: Independent Practitioners Win Direct Payment—With No M.D.-Strings Attached." *RN* 41: 11–12.

Sifton, David W., ed. "Nursing News: Plan Pays Same Fee for M.D., R.N. Care." *RN* 41:7.

Sifton, David W., ed. "Nursing News: Study Advocates Equal Pay for Nurse Practitioner and M.D. Doing Same Work." *RN* 41: 25.

Simchuk, Cathy J., R.N. "Development of Criteria for Emergency Department Nursing Audit." *Journal of Emergency Nursing* 3: 47–49.

Simms, Elsie. "Preparation for Independent Practice." *Nursing Outlook* 25: 114–118.

Skipper, James K., Jr. "Addendum to the Right to Adequate Health Care." *Nursing Digest* 4: 17–18.

Smith, Hilary. "What Do Nurses Do In America?" *American Journal of Nursing* 76: 278–280.

"Social Security Amendments of 1972." *United States Code Congressional and Administrative News.* Volume 1. West Publishing Company, October 30, 1972, pp. 1548–1747.

Stanley, Linda, R.N., B.S.N. " 'Expanded-Role' Nursing Hits the Hospitals." *RN* 41: 54–59.

Stone, Sandra, M.S.; Berger, Marie Strang, M.S.; Elhart, Dorothy, M.S.; Firsich, Cannell Sharon, M.S.; and Jordan, Shelly Baney, M.N. *Management for Nurses.* St. Louis: The C. V. Mosby Company, 1976.

Subrin, Lawrence I., C.P.A. "The Business Aspects of Private Nursing Practice." *Journal of Nursing Administration* 7: 12–13, 50–51.

Tate, Curtis E., Jr.; Megginson, Leon C.; Scott, Charles R., Jr.; and Trueblood, Lyle R. *The Complete Guide to Your Own Business.* Homewood, Illinois: Dow Jones-Irwin, 1977.

Taylor, Ann Gill, R.N., M.S., Ed.D. "Decision-Making in Nursing." *Imprint* 25: 50–51, 68–9.

Thompson, Edward T., ed. "News From the World of Medicine: Not So Private Files." *Reader's Digest* 110: 35.

Trager, Brahna. "Home Care: Providing the Right to Stay Home." *Hospitals JAHA* 49: 98.

Trout, M. D., M.D., J.D., F.C.L.M. "New York State Malpractice Legislation." *The Journal of Legal Medicine* 3: 16–7.

Ubell, Earl. "The Great American Health Insurance Machine, Part II." *Family Health* 10: 46–48.

Ubell, Earl. "Unraveling the Mysteries of Health Insurance, Part I." *Family Health* 10: 22–25, 27.

Uustal, Diane B. "Values Clarification in Nursing: Application to Practice." *American Journal of Nursing* 78: 2058–63.

Van Nostrand, Lymann G., M.P.A. "Capital Financing for Health Facilities." *Public Health Reports* 92: 499–507.

Vengroski, Stella M., R.N., M.A. and Saarman, Lembi, R.N., M.S. "Peer Review in Quality Assurance." *American Journal of Nursing* 78: 2094–6.

Vogl, A.J., ed. "Practice Management: If a Certified Termination Letter Isn't Claimed." *Medical Economics,* September 5, 1977, pp. 55–56.

Vogl, A. J., ed. "The Father of Medicare Looks at National Health Insurance." *Medical Economics,* September 5, 1977, pp. 219–226.

Watkins, Robert. "Health Insurance for All in Three Years—or so Says Senator Kennedy." *Modern Medicine* 43: 14, 16.

Wehr, Elizabeth. "Carter Lists 'Principles' of National Health Plan." *Congressional Quarterly Weekly Report* 36: 2058–9.

Wehr, Elizabeth. "Dilemma Over National Health Insurance Delays Promised Carter Plan." *Congressional Quarterly Weekly Report* 36: 1770–3.

Wehr, Elizabeth. "Senate Defies Carter on Nurse Training Aid." *Congressional Quarterly Weekly Report* 36: 1544–5.

Welch, Cathryne A. "Health Care Distribution and Third-Party Payment for Nurses' Services." *American Journal of Nursing* 75: 1844–1847.

Wentzel, Marcela L. "Family Reactions to Parental Institutionalization." *Nursing Homes* 27: 6–8.

Young, Katherine Jean, R.N., M.N. "Independent Nurse Practitioner: Concept of Practice." *Nurse Practitioner* 2: 10–12.

Young, Katherine Jean, R.N. "Independent Nurse Practitioner: The Practical Issues of Practice." *Nurse Practitioner* 2: 14–17.

Zornow, Ruth Ann. "A Curriculum Model for the Expanded Role." *Nursing Outlook* 25: 43–46.

Index